Brain Stimulation Therapies
FOR CLINICIANS

SECOND EDITION

Brain Stimulation Therapies
FOR CLINICIANS
SECOND EDITION

by

Edmund S. Higgins, M.D.
Mark S. George, M.D.

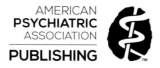

AMERICAN
PSYCHIATRIC
ASSOCIATION
PUBLISHING
™

If you wish to buy 50 or more copies of the same title, please go to www.appi.org/specialdiscounts for more information.

Copyright © 2020 American Psychiatric Association Publishing

ALL RIGHTS RESERVED

Second Edition

Manufactured in the United States of America on acid-free paper
23 22 21 20 19   5 4 3 2 1

American Psychiatric Association Publishing
800 Maine Avenue SW
Suite 900
Washington, DC 20024-2812
www.appi.org

Library of Congress Cataloging-in-Publication Data
Names: Higgins, Edmund S., author. | George, Mark S. (Mark Stork), author. | American Psychiatric Association Publishing, publisher.
Title: Brain stimulation therapies for clinicians / by Edmund S. Higgins, Mark S. George.
Description: Second edition. | Washington, D.C. : American Psychiatric Association Publishing, [2020] | Includes bibliographical references and index.
Identifiers: LCCN 2019019784 (print) | LCCN 2019021764 (ebook) | ISBN 9781615372706 (ebook) | ISBN 9781615371679 (hardcover : alk. paper)
Subjects: | MESH: Electric Stimulation Therapy | Electroconvulsive Therapy | Deep Brain Stimulation
Classification: LCC RC350.B72 (ebook) | LCC RC350.B72 (print) | NLM WB 495 | DDC 616.89/122—dc23
LC record available at https://lccn.loc.gov/2019019784

British Library Cataloguing in Publication Data
A CIP record is available from the British Library.

Contents

About the Authors vii

Foreword to the First Edition ix
Michael Trimble, M.D., F.R.C.P., F.R.C.Psych.

Preface to the Second Edition xiii

Acknowledgments. xvii

Glossary xix

1 Introduction 1

2 Basic Electricity 13

3 Electrical Brain 31

4 Electroconvulsive Therapy 45

5 Vagus Nerve Stimulation 71

6 Transcranial Magnetic Stimulation. 95

7 Deep Brain Stimulation and
Cortical Stimulation 121

8 Transcranial Direct Current Stimulation 147

9 Other Techniques. 159

10 Future Techniques 169

Appendix by Disease 179

Appendix by Stimulation Method 181

Index 183

About the Authors

Edmund S. Higgins, M.D., is a Clinical Associate Professor of Family Medicine and Psychiatry at the Medical University of South Carolina (MUSC). He received his medical degree from Case Western Reserve University School of Medicine. He completed residencies in Family Practice and Psychiatry at MUSC. He has a private psychiatric practice and is a staff psychiatrist for the South Carolina Department of Corrections. He lives on Sullivan's Island, South Carolina.

Mark S. George, M.D., is a Distinguished Professor of Psychiatry, Radiology, and Neuroscience, as well as director of the Brain Stimulation Laboratory and former director of the Center for Advanced Imaging Research, at the Medical University of South Carolina, Charleston. He received his medical degree and completed dual residencies at MUSC in both neurology and psychiatry and is board certified in both areas. After a fellowship in London in 1989, where he first encountered transcranial magnetic stimulation, and four years at the National Institute of Mental Health in Bethesda, Maryland, he returned to Charleston, where he has conducted pioneering work with functional imaging of the brain and several of the brain stimulation techniques, particularly TMS and vagus nerve stimulation. He is on several editorial review boards, has published over 500 scientific articles or book chapters, holds eight patents, and has written or edited four books, including a previous book in collaboration with Dr. Higgins. Dr. George is the editor-in-chief of *Brain Stimulation: Basic, Translational and Clinical Research in Neuromodulation*. He too resides on Sullivan's Island, South Carolina.

Disclosure of Competing Interests

Edmund S. Higgins, M.D., has no competing interests to disclose.

Mark S. George, M.D., has no equity ownership in any device or pharmaceutical company. His total industry compensation is less than 10% of university salary. Medical University of South Carolina has filed six patents or invention disclosures in Dr. George's name regarding brain imaging and stimulation.

Foreword to the First Edition

Michael Trimble, M.D., F.R.C.P., F.R.C.Psych.

One of the most important neuroscience discoveries of the twentieth century, or perhaps of all time, arguably was that of Olds and Milner in the early 1950s (Olds 1973). For centuries, the brain had been viewed as a passive recipient of sensory impressions, which led in a Pavlov-type sequence to motor action, with, in some (behavioralist) philosophies, the assumption that little of relevance occurred between stimulus and response. And yet a growing undercurrent of knowledge was emphasizing the prepared brain, the brain not as a receptacle and *tabula rasa* but as an active organ, a synthesizing and creating brain. Proceeding from the philosophies of Kant and Nietzsche and the psychologies of Freud and his successors, the very drivenness of human activity, by unconscious and in some theories unknowable forces, became common currency. But these hollow frames lacked a neurological framework, a neurobiology of the emotions and movement.

What Olds and Milner did was uncover cerebral circuits for pleasure and reward, endowing hedonic tone to percepts and behavior. This research was being conducted at the same time that others, notably Papez and MacLean, were unraveling additional neuroanatomical structures associated with the emotions. Papez (1937) proposed a circuit for emotion, giving an organism a "stream of feeling." MacLean (1990) defined for us the "visceral" brain. The latter was renamed *limbic* after the earlier anatomical designa-

---

Prof. Trimble is Emeritus Professor in Behavioural Neurology at the Institute of Neurology, University College, London.

tions of Broca, and the term *limbic system* is now familiar to all neuroscientists with an interest in brain-behavior relationships.

With the identification of such a neuroanatomy of the emotions, the possibility emerged of altering emotional expression and hence providing amelioration of neurobehavioral disturbances by influencing such circuitry. Stimulation of the brain, whether indirectly across the scalp or directly by application of electrodes to the brain itself, could be realized. In fact, such ideas had been around for a long time, but the neuroanatomical knowledge and the technology were not available until the mid-twentieth century. One well-acknowledged method, still widely used, was electroconvulsive therapy (ECT). Exactly how it worked to lyse a psychosis or cure a melancholia was and remains unclear.

As is reviewed in the introductory chapter of this book, the early pioneers of direct stimulation had the right ideas but lacked the sophistication that today's electronic world has provided. Robert Heath (1954) was one such investigator. While at Tulane, Heath began stimulation of what he referred to as the "septal area" (closely analogous to what is also referred to as the *fundus striati*, loosely, the accumbens region), in patients with schizophrenia. The choice of target was interesting, given that the subcortical controls over the cortex, and therefore behavior, were implicated in his theories (he also stimulated the caudate, thalamus, hypothalamus, and cerebellum). Since patients were usually conscious, their subjective responses could be recorded. These included sensations of pleasure, akin to the findings in animal models of Olds and Milner.

There was one important snag in the animal studies, which interfered with the investigations, namely that some of the animals developed epileptic seizures and died. This experimental artifact was seized upon by Graham Goddard (1967), who recognized it as a possible model for the "kindling" of long-lasting changes of excitability in cerebral circuits, and as a possible experimental model of epilepsy.

The clinical work on treating major psychiatric disorders and abnormal movements by lesioning subcortical structures was quite successful, but the amount of operative tissue destruction that occurred often led to unwanted neuropsychological deficits. In any case, a new era of treatment evolved with the discovery of the modes of action of monoamine transmitters, especially dopamine, and the development of an array of neuropsychoactive drugs, the success of which soon diminished enthusiasm for the neurosurgery to treat neuropsychiatric disorders.

On account of the development of new methods of brain stimulation, there is now a renaissance of interest in reevaluating the data from the early studies, in part to assess the most relevant neuronal structures for targets. Such information is guiding neurosurgical methods for deep brain stimulation (DBS) and is helping to reformulate hypotheses about the mechanisms of action of ECT and other stimulation techniques that have become available or that will be available in the near future. It is to these theories and to these techniques that this book is directed. If progress in this area is as rapid as it has been in the past few years, some form of brain stimulation will be a treatment modality—some may predict *the* treatment modality—for a wide variety of neurological and psychiatric disorders. Acquaintance with the basic principles of electricity will be essential for all providers who work in this field, as is an understanding of, say, serotonin or dopamine today. Discussing treatment options with patients will necessitate an understanding of neuroanatomy, an explanation of the methods of action of various stimulation techniques, and the benefits and hazards of the options.

To these ends, this book is timely and important. Starting at the beginning (with history), the current *olla podrida* of brain stimulation techniques along with their supposed mechanisms of action are reviewed in a language that is clear and jargon-free. There is clearly much to learn, but progress is fast. Soon, implanted devices will be able to predict the onset of seizures and target pulses to stop them from evolving, treat a wide spectrum of movement disorders, and alter the progression of major psychopathologies, with little apparent problem with either compliance or significant side effects. I predict that a succession of revised versions will follow from this first edition of the book, and that even the authors will look back with surprise that they had not more accurately predicted the future.

References

Goddard GV: Development of epileptic seizures through brain stimula-
    tion at low intensity. Nature 214:1020–1021, 1967
Heath RG: Studies in Schizophrenia: A Multi-Disciplinary Approach to
    Mind-Brain Relationships. Cambridge, MA, Harvard University
    Press, 1954
MacLean PD: The Triune Brain in Evolution. New York, Plenum, 1990
Olds J: The discovery of reward systems in the brain, in Brain Stimula-
    tion and Motivation: Research and Commentary. Edited by Elliot
    Valenstein. Glenview, IL, Scott Foresman, 1973
Papez JW: A proposed mechanism of emotion. Arch Neurol Psychiatry
    38:725–743, 1937

Preface to the Second Edition

The field of brain stimulation is exploding with research activity across basic and clinical domains. Currently, at least 13 forms of brain stimulation are undergoing development and evaluation as interventions for neurological and psychiatric disorders. Stimulation techniques are a unique form of treatment distinctly different from pharmacology, psychotherapy, or physical therapy. While the developments in this burgeoning field are exciting, the amount of information can be overwhelming for practicing clinicians as well as patients. This book should serve as an overview of the brain stimulation therapies for anyone seeking a broad grasp of the field.

The brain stimulation therapies range from noninvasive techniques, such as transcranial magnetic stimulation (TMS), which applies single or repetitive stimuli at the scalp surface, to more invasive techniques, such as deep brain stimulation (DBS), which involves neurosurgical implantation of electrodes in specific brain regions. These interventions differ in many fundamental characteristics, such as whether stimulation results in seizures or is nonconvulsive, is continuous or intermittent, or uses brain activity to determine the timing or site of stimulation.

The brain stimulation techniques thus represent a new class of therapeutics that has already displayed remarkable potential for producing novel therapeutic effects. For example, DBS for Parkinson's disease produces symptom remission almost instantly in patients whose symptoms largely are refractory to all medications. These therapeutic effects continue in many patients for up to 15 years. These remarkable therapeutic effects may arise because the focal brain stimulation methods trigger therapeutic mechanisms different from those that follow from medications.

Related to this difference in approach, the side effects of the brain stimulation techniques also differ radically from those of conventional treatments like medications or medical interventions. All the forms of focal brain stimulation reviewed in this book involve the passage of an electrical current through neural tissue, either peripherally or centrally. However in general, electricity has no metabolite or other residue. Thus, the therapeutic and adverse effects of these interventions are largely determined by the endogenous or adaptive response of the brain to the electrical stimulation. In this sense, these methods are perhaps more "natural" than some other forms of therapy, although external electricity is not exactly natural. The brain stimulation therapies are thus creating another therapeutic option or class, complementing talking therapies, medications, and rehabilitation, and in some cases replacing ablative surgery.

Anyone who is not daily working in this field can be stymied by all the new information when confronted with a patient who might benefit from one of the brain stimulation techniques. As with genetics or brain imaging, there is an initially daunting "acronym soup" that can hinder access and cause confusion. This book tries to provide a clear and straightforward analysis of the prevailing techniques, and in some sense is an elaborate dictionary for these acronyms and the new methods. The book starts with a quick overview of electricity and physics—elements common to all the methods but that are not taught in medical school. We review the relevant neuroanatomy, physics, and methods for each technique. We then critically and efficiently review the clinical literature for each method. This book is thus intended to be a quick first start, helping clinicians, patients, and researchers efficiently understand the current knowledge about the techniques. As is often found in any new area of technology or medicine, there are some who falsely advocate certain techniques and claim therapeutic effects for which there is little or no supporting evidence. We have tried to impartially separate the "wheat" from the "chaff" so that everyone can quickly have the latest data at their fingertips and then decide for themselves.

Readers of this book should gain a good understanding of the current state of brain stimulation therapies. This can then be used to help patients and provide the background for keeping up with this rapidly evolving and most exciting field.

We hope that you enjoy reading this book and find the contents "stimulating" and helpful. It was a labor of love for us, and we hope a similar response will be induced in the readers.

Edmund S. Higgins, M.D.
Mark S. George, M.D.

Acknowledgments

From E.S.H.

I want to thank Cindy Andrews for assistance with the figures in this book. This book is easier on the eyes because of her input. It was her suggestion to use the outline of a nineteenth-century female portrait as the model for the different stimulation techniques. This suggestion has added a humanistic perspective to what can often be portrayed as technological and futuristic.

I also wish to thank my son Grady Higgins, who produced Figures 2–1 and 7–7 on various Tuesday mornings before the start of school.

From M.S.G.

I would like to acknowledge the pioneers of electricity, Ben Franklin, Nikola Tesla, Thomas Edison, and George Westinghouse, without whom we would not have the external power sources for the brain stimulation techniques.

I feel a need to acknowledge the early pioneers of brain localization and brain stimulation techniques, such as John Hughlings Jackson, James Crichton-Browne, David Ferrier, and Charles Sherrington. These were the initial pioneers of many of the techniques discussed in this book. I would personally like to thank Dr. Michael Trimble, who first introduced me to their writings and ideas when I worked in London.

There have been many people who have helped me with my ideas and interests in brain imaging and brain stimulation, both skeptics and advocates. Thanks to friends and colleagues in both groups, and especially those who started in one and then moved to the other based on scientific data. James Ballenger, Robert Post, Tom Uhde, Harold Sackeim, Thomas Schlaepfer, Saxby Pridmore, Mark Hallett, and Eric Wassermann have all gone far out of their way to teach, encourage, or facilitate my understanding of these techniques. I would especially like to thank my friend and colleague of the last decade, Ziad Nahas, who has a wealth of ideas and energy concerning this field.

I would like to thank my family for their help and support over the years, especially for not discouraging me when I was pursuing some "out of the box" brain stimulation research—my sisters Bebe and Jane and their families, for not freaking out the Christmas evening when I showed up with a scalp abrasion from some TMS studies; and my ex-wife Eloise, and my two children, Laura and Daniel, who grew up in and around MRI scanners and stimulation laboratories.

However, I am especially grateful to one group in particular. Those are the patients who have participated in clinical trials and have helped me and the field learn what works and what does not. Without their "leap of faith" participation in double-blind studies, we would get nowhere. Thanks. We dedicate this book to all of you.

Glossary

Acronym/ Name	Full name
CBS	Cortical brain stimulation
CES	Cranial electrotherapy stimulation
DBS	Deep brain stimulation
ECT	Electroconvulsive therapy
EEG	Electroencephalography
Electroshock	*See* ECT
EPI-fMRI	Echoplanar imaging functional MRI
FEAST	Focal electrically applied seizure therapy
FEAT	Focal electrically applied therapy
fMRI	Functional magnetic resonance imaging
MEG	Magnetoencephalography
MENS	Microcurrent electrical neuromuscular stimulation
MRI	Magnetic resonance imaging
MST	Magnetic seizure therapy
PET	Positron emission tomography
PTNS	Percutaneous tibial nerve stimulation
RNS	Responsive neural stimulation
RST	Responsive stimulation therapy
rTMS	Repetitive transcranial magnetic stimulation
Shock therapy	*See* ECT
SNS	Sacral nerve stimulation
tACS	Transcranial alternating current stimulation
tDCS	Transcranial direct current stimulation
TENS	Transcutaneous electrical nerve stimulation
tLVMAS	Transcutaneous low-voltage microamperage stimulation
TMS	Transcranial magnetic stimulation
tRNS	Transcranial random noise stimulation
VNS	Vagus nerve stimulation

CHAPTER 1

Introduction

The human brain is perhaps the most complex organ known to exist in the universe. One hundred billion neurons with 100 trillion connections sense, analyze, and respond to the environment in ways that are beyond our current comprehension. Ostensibly, it all boils down to electrical and chemical communication. Figure 1–1 shows the stereotypical synapse that highlights the electrical and chemical nature of one neuron communicating with another.

Historically, neurologists have been more aware of the electrical nature of the brain, whereas psychiatrists, until just recently, have concentrated almost exclusively on the neurotransmitters and psychopharmacology. Psychiatry had become so enamored with neurotransmitters that "chemical imbalance" became part of our common language. Some patients think it is an actual diagnosis.

Electro

1. The action potential arrives at the presynaptic terminal.

2. Depolarization causes voltage-gated calcium channels to open and results in a large influx of Ca^{2+}.

3. Exocytosis: Ca^{2+} causes the vesicles to fuse with the membrane and release the neurotransmitter.

4. Excitatory postsynaptic potentials (EPSP) spread out over the dendrite.

Chemical

A. Precursor molecules and enzymes are transported down the axon from the cell body along the microtubules.

B. Enzymes in the synaptic terminal convert the precursor molecules into active neurotransmitter.

C. The neurotransmitter is stored in the vesicles until released by the influx of Ca^{2+}.

D. The released neurotransmitter binds with the receptors on the post-synaptic terminal and generates an EPSP.

E. Reuptake of the neurotransmitter limits the duration of the signal and allows the cell to recycle the neuro-transmitter.

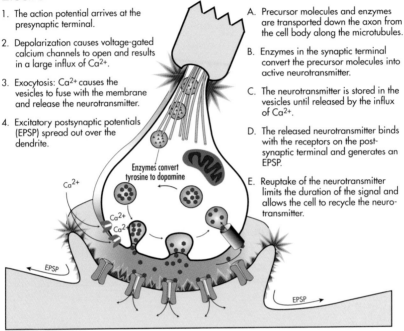

FIGURE 1-1.　Electrochemical communication.
Communication between two neurons in the brain includes both electrical and chemical mechanisms, which are linked. The electrical impulse becomes a chemical messenger, which then converts the information back into an electrical signal.
Source.　Adapted from Higgins and George 2007.

We believe electricity is the currency of the brain. Although chemical and electrical features are in fact different features of looking at the same process, and neurotransmitters are essential to conduct information, it is the electricity that does the heavy lifting. Hopefully, clinicians in the future will be more adept at recognizing the importance of both the electrical and the chemical features of each patient's problems.

　　Brain stimulation, unlike pharmacology, focuses on the electrical mechanisms of the brain, which then cause localized changes in pharmacology. Applications of electrical stimulation through a variety of new and old techniques can correct underlying disorders. Traditionally, brain stimulation therapies have been highly invasive and reserved for those individuals with treatment-resistant disorders. However, there are a variety of new brain stimulation treatments that are neither invasive nor solely for the severely impaired. More and more researchers are wondering if brain stimulation can augment normal performance—for example, improve academic retention, enhance video game performance, or potentially even help someone win an Olympic medal. (The data are controversial and underwhelming at this time, but the future is wide open.)

Brain stimulation therapies are treatment options that have grown over the past few decades and will continue to grow in the coming years. New delivery mechanisms and wider applications of existing technologies are clearly in the future of central nervous system (CNS) treatments. The goal of this book is to bring a greater understanding of the field to practicing clinicians (neurologists, psychiatrists, psychologists, nurses, other health professionals). Before we get into the details of brain stimulation therapies, however, let us review some of the pioneers who brought us to this point.

History of Electrical Stimulation

Live fish were perhaps the earliest brain stimulation devices. The ancient Greeks and Romans knew of the shocking powers of the Nile catfish and electric ray (Finger 2000). Galen and Scribonius Largus in Rome used electric rays to treat headaches and various other disorders (Figure 1–2). They placed the fish across the brow of a suffering patient or had the patient stand on several live rays. The fish were allowed to discharge their special powers, which, of course, were not recognized as electricity until many centuries later. Unfortunately, electric rays were not readily available, and it is not clear whether these interventions helped or simply satisfied the human urge to *do something*. It was not until the eighteenth century that machines were created that could produce electricity on demand.

By the early eighteenth century, the leading scientists of the time still did not know what substance was flowing through nerves (Finger 2000). Serious thinkers speculated about spirits, special fluids, and even vibrations. It was Luigi Galvani who, in

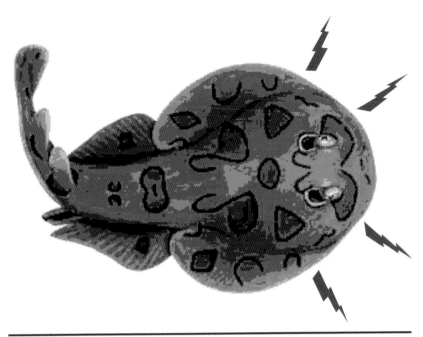

FIGURE 1–2.   Early brain stimulation device.

Electric rays are arguably the first brain stimulation devices. They were used by the ancient Greeks and Romans to treat various disorders.

a series of experiments published in 1791, established that electricity flows through nerves. Using rudimentary batteries, he showed that an exposed nerve could be activated with electricity and produce a seemingly natural muscle contraction. Furthermore, he established that nature's own electricity (e.g., lightning) produced a similar response to electrical machines.

Macabre Research

Aldini, Galvani's devoted nephew, conducted some of the most unusual research and showed that human muscles also moved when electrically stimulated. He applied electricity to decapitated heads at the base of a guillotine and was able to induce jaw movements, grimaces, and eye openings.

Motor Cortex

The discovery of the motor cortex was the next great example of the importance of electricity to CNS activity (Finger 2000). Gustav Fritsch noticed during the Prusso-Danish War that accidentally irritating exposed brains of head-injured soldiers often resulted in a twitch to the opposite side of the body. In the late 1860s Fritsch teamed up with Eduard Hitzig, a German physician. Together they systematically explored the cortex of dogs. Their success in identifying the motor cortex lay in gentle electrical stimulation of the cortex. Apparently, they would touch the electrode to their tongues to determine the appropriate current before stimulating the dog's cortex.

Charles Sherrington in the early 1900s continued mapping out the details of the motor cortex. Using lightly anesthetized apes and monkeys, he was the first to recognize the contiguous nature of the motor control along the cortex. It was the great Canadian neurosurgeon Wilder Penfield who, along with others, extended Sherrington's work and delineated the odd-shaped little man (the motor homunculus) embedded in the cortex (Penfield 1968) (Figure 1–3).

Epilepsy Surgery

In the 1930s, Penfield explored the human brain in live epilepsy patients as part of the surgical excision of the epileptic focus of the seizures (Lewis 1983). Penfield was having more success at the surgical treatment for intractable seizures than had previously been found. Part of his success came from a thorough exploration of the cortex in the patients who remained awake with their brain exposed under local anesthesia. Penfield's goal was to locate the focus of the seizure activity, generally known from the symptoms at the start of the seizure. Once the focus was located, Penfield worked to remove the damaged tissue while preserving as much normal brain function as possible.

To stimulate the patient's cortex, Penfield used a probe with weak electrical activity (and he never touched it to his tongue, as far as we know). Because the patients were awake, they could describe what they experienced, which facilitated the differentia-

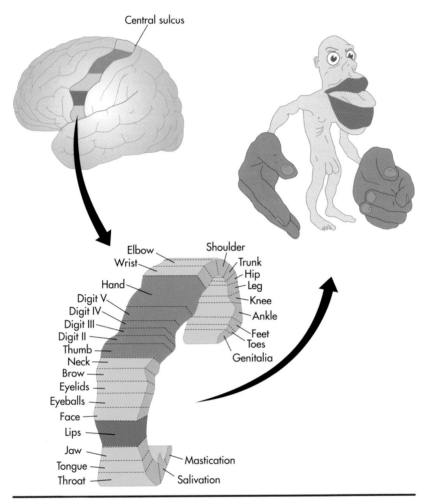

FIGURE 1–3. The motor cortex and motor homunculus.

Source.   Adapted from Rosenzweig et al. 2005.

tion of diseased from normal brain tissue. One of the interesting findings from this work were the reactions some patients experienced with temporal lobe stimulation. While stimulating many regions of the brain (e.g., occipital cortex, motor cortex, Broca's area) generated predictable responses, the findings from the temporal lobes were unexpected.

Stimulation of the temporal lobes sometimes generated memories of distant events from the patients' lives. Some remembered experiences from childhood; others heard songs they had not remembered in many years. The memories would stop when the stimulation terminated and sometimes could be replicated with a second stimulation. These findings introduced the belief that the long-sought-after *memory engram* had been found. The thinking went something like this: memory entails the storage of an experience, and Penfield had discovered the neural representation of the memory (the memory engram). The finding was widely repeated and for a while was dogma in introductory psychology textbooks, but it has since lost favor. It has never been clear that what the patients recalled were actual memories; less than 10% of the patients who received temporal lobe stimulation reported a memory, and often the memories were associated with the aura from the intractable seizure that Penfield was trying to find and remove.

Transcranial magnetic stimulation (TMS) can induce sensations from the occipital cortex, motor cortex, and Broca's area similar to what is found with direct electrical stimulation. TMS does this by inducing an electrical impulse (more on this later). However, TMS over the temporal lobes does not seem to produce memories similar to what Penfield found, further evidence that Penfield did not discover the repository of our memories.

Memory Engram

The idea that we can store all our memories in a physical form that can be retrieved at some very distant time has an undeniable romantic appeal. Psychologists now believe we only store bits and pieces of memories, which we reconstruct to recall our past—the way a dinosaur is reconstructed from bone fragments. However, memories must leave some physical trace in the brain, and the race continues to find the engram.

Self-Stimulation

Brain stimulation allows exploration of the function of parts of the brain. When exciting the cortex, stimulation is the opposite of lesioning a site. Self-stimulation enables researchers to explore reward and punishment circuits in animals who are otherwise unable to describe the effects of the electrical stimulation. Work by James Olds and Peter Milner at McGill University transformed the field with their accidental discovery in 1954.

Olds and Milner were studying brain stimulation of the reticular formation and the effects this would have on alertness and learning (Olds 1956). As part of the study, Olds and Milner wanted to be sure that stimulation of the electrode was not an adverse experience for the rat. Much to their amazement, the rat seemed to like the stimulation. Apparently, one of the electrodes accidentally bent when placed in the rat's brain and ended up in an unexpected location.

When the rat was allowed to self-stimulate with a Skinner Box arrangement (Figure 1–4), the results were even more striking. Some rats would self-stimulate 2,000 times an hour for 24 hours. Hungry rats would self-stimulate before eating available food. Olds and Milner had discovered that the brain contains circuits for reward, or what some call "pleasure centers." This has led to recognition of reward centers in the brain, which are present to enhance species survival (e.g., eating, sex, power) but also can be usurped by drugs of abuse or naughty behaviors.

Emotional Pacemaker

In the early 1950s, Robert Heath, chairman of psychiatry at Tulane University in New Orleans, worked with neurosurgeons to implant electrodes in psychiatric patients with severe, unremitting disorders. The research was not fruitful. However, the discoveries by Olds and Milner stirred Heath to pursue stimulation of deep cortical structures associated with pleasure as a potential treatment for depression, intractable pain, schizophrenia, or homosexuality.

Heath believed that anhedonia is the basic underlying problem for many psychiatric conditions (Valenstein 1973). That is, an inability to experience pleasure is an integral part of the disorder. He hoped that stimulation of the pleasure circuits would reawaken dormant neural pathways and result in improved mood, interest, and energy. Heath and others believed that a regimen of brain

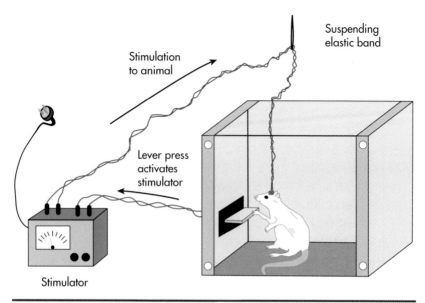

FIGURE 1–4.   In pursuit of stimulation.

Olds and Milner utilized a Skinner Box to study the propensity of rats to seek electrical self-stimulation.

stimulation could be conceptualized as an "emotional pacemaker" for patients with serious mental disorders.

Although ahead of his time, Heath ultimately abandoned this line of research. He was disappointed with the lack of long-term benefits. Typically, the positive results quickly diminished after the stimulation was turned off. Likewise, he was working at a time when the equipment available was cumbersome and not portable.

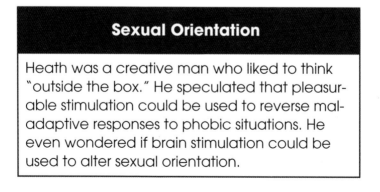

Sexual Orientation

Heath was a creative man who liked to think "outside the box." He speculated that pleasurable stimulation could be used to reverse maladaptive responses to phobic situations. He even wondered if brain stimulation could be used to alter sexual orientation.

> ## Sexual Orientation *(continued)*
>
> It was a time when homosexuality was seen as a disorder. Heath implanted an electrode in a young man with a long history of psychiatric problems, including depression and substance dependence, who was also homosexual (Moan and Heath 1972). He then recruited a New Orleans sex worker to engage the patient in heterosexual intercourse while the patient simultaneously received pleasurable brain stimulation. Although the patient was able to enjoy heterosexual activity during the experimental session and afterward, it is unclear if the intervention changed his sexual orientation or diminished his psychiatric problems.
>
> The experiment caused much controversy, was not well regarded in the medical community, and has never been repeated.

Brain Chips

José Delgado, a professor of physiology at Yale, was one of the other great pioneers of brain stimulation (Horgan 2005). He too had participated in implanting electrodes during the 1950s, but he took the field one step further. He developed and implanted radio-equipped electrodes, which he called "stimoreceivers." Using cats, monkeys, apes, and even humans, he was able to remotely stimulate a device as small as a half-dollar completely implanted in the brain.

Delgado's most impressive experiments involved brain stimulation to inhibit aggressive behavior. In one particularly dramatic demonstration, Delgado stood in the ring with a charging bull. With the press of one button, Delgado brought the bull to a dead stop just a few feet in front of him.

Delgado's work was troubling to many people. The idea of controlling behavior with technology seemed like mind control administered by a totalitarian dictator. Of interest, Delgado also received a number of requests from psychotic patients who wanted him to remove the transmitter they believed was in their brain, controlling their thoughts. Fortunately, brain stimulation, and the focus of this book, has been used to reduce suffering rather than control behavior.

Conclusions

It is clear from this brief review of the history of brain stimulation that there really are no new ideas under the sun. Several pioneering scientists foreshadowed the current use of brain stimulation at a time when psychiatry was dominated by psychoanalytic thinking. This was a time even before the pharmacological revolution.

There were several disadvantages working against these early pioneers. They had more primitive and bulky technology with which to work. Additionally, they had limited understanding of the important brain structures. More than 30 years of brain imaging have now yielded a much better understanding of regional functional neuroanatomy.

Beginning with these meager seeds, the field of brain stimulation is now a fertile maturing tree with several branches. Our goal in this book is to acquaint you with an overview of the current status of the field.

References

Finger S: Minds Behind the Brain: A History of the Pioneers and Their Discoveries. New York, Oxford University Press, 2000

Higgins ES, George MS: The Neuroscience of Clinical Psychiatry: The Pathophysiology of Behavior and Mental Illness. Baltimore, MD, Lippincott, Williams & Wilkins, 2007

Horgan J: The forgotten era of brain chips. Sci Am 293(4):66–73, 2005 16196255

Lewis J: Something Hidden: A Biography of Wilder Penfield. Halifax, Nova Scotia, Goodread Biographies, 1983

Moan CE, Heath RG: Septal stimulation for the initiation of heterosexual behavior in a homosexual male. J Behav Ther Exp Psychiatry 3(1):23–30, 1972

Olds J: Pleasure centers in the brain. Sci Am 195(4):105–117, 1956

Penfield W: Engrams in the human brain. Mechanisms of memory. Proc R Soc Med 61(8):831–840, 1968 4299804

Rosenzweig MR, Breedlove SM, Watson NV: Biological Psychology, 4th Edition. Sunderland, MA, Sinauer, 2005

Valenstein ES: Brain Control: A Critical Examination of Brain Stimulation and Psychosurgery. New York, John Wiley and Sons, 1973

CHAPTER 2

Basic Electricity

Overview of Electricity

Electricity is one of the fundamental forces of nature. Brain stimulation involves applying focal harnessed electrical power back into the central nervous system (CNS). In this chapter, we review the basic principles of electricity to gain a better understanding of what is being applied in brain stimulation. Chapter 3 discusses what actually happens in the brain naturally with electricity and when we apply it externally.

Electrons

Electrical current is the flow of electrons. Atoms are made up of protons, neutrons, and electrons (Figure 2–1). The protons and neutrons in the nucleus are held together with nuclear forces. The protons are positively charged, while the neutrons are neutral. The electrons spinning around the outside of the atom are negatively charged. The positive charge on the protons attracts the negatively charged electrons and keeps the atom electrically neutral. Atoms can lose or gain electrons. It is the movement of negatively charged electrons that constitutes an electrical current.

Electrons need a force to coax them to move. "Electrical pressure" is needed to make electrons flow in a wire. Electrical pressure is a force called *electromotive force,* or **voltage**. An easy way to understand this is to compare electricity to plumbing. The current of electrons moving through a wire is like water moving through a pipe. The electromotive force needed to move the electrons is like the drop in elevation (gravity) that makes the water flow down the pipe.

Direct Current

Understanding how a battery can generate a direct current is a good way to refresh our understanding of electricity. When electrons move in one direction, it is called a *direct current.* A battery, or *dry cell*, provides one method to get electrons moving through a wire in the same direction.

A battery is basically two different metals in an electrolyte solution. Most metals have a propensity to give away electrons and become more positively charged. Some metals have a greater propensity to give up electrons than others. Two metals, one more willing to give up electrons and the other more willing to accept electrons, can create an electromotive force. The key is placing them in an electrolyte mixture where the electrons can be moved from one metal to the other so that they can flow.

Figure 2–2 shows an example of this process. Electrons tend to leave copper and move toward zinc. These electrons flow through the electrolyte solution ammonium chloride in a process that is beyond the scope of this text. The buildup of electrons on the zinc

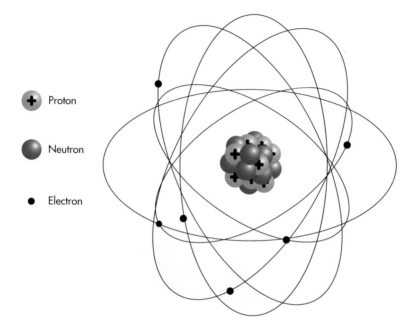

Proton

Neutron

Electron

FIGURE 2-1. A simple atom.

An atom is composed of protons, neutrons, and electrons. The flow of electrons from one atom to another is the essential component of electricity.

terminal creates electrical pressure. The potential electrical pressure is measured in **volts**—in this case, about 1.1 volts.

The wire connecting the copper terminal and the zinc terminal allows electrons to move back in the direction of the gradient—like water flowing downhill. The movement of the electrons is the **current**, which heats up the filament in the light bulb and generates light. This process will continue until the copper has been eaten away or the electrolyte evaporates. **Thus, the pressure is voltage, and the flow is current.** These are related but different. Current, measured in *amperes*, is the amount of charge (measured in *coulombs*) flowing through something over time. In Figure 2–2, the light bulb is the resistance in the system. This brings us to an important element of understanding electricity—**Ohm's law**.

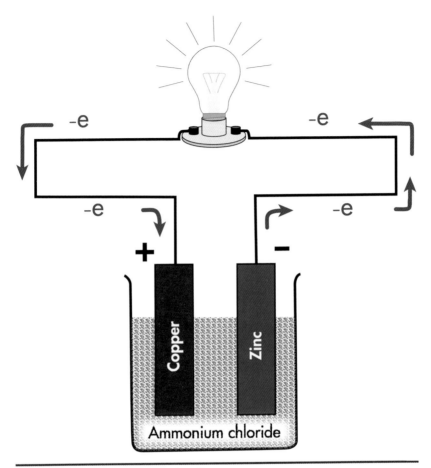

FIGURE 2–2. A simple battery.

In a chemical process, electrons move from the copper to the zinc in the ammonium chloride. This creates an electrical potential. The wire enables the electrons to move back to the copper, creating an electrical circuit and powering the light.

The current (flow, or I) is the same as the pressure (voltage, or V) divided by the resistance (R): $I = (V/R)$. You can thus increase current by increasing the voltage (pressure) or dropping the resistance. Another important term is the **current density**, which is the amount of current in a specific area. High current densities can be toxic to nerve cells and thus are a limiting aspect of most brain stimulation methods.

In Figure 2–2, knowing Ohm's law, we can set up the system to where the pressure stays the same regardless of what happens in the light bulb (constant voltage), or we can have it adapt to the full system and always provide the same flow (constant current). Interestingly, the different brain stimulation techniques have used each of these approaches, and they produce markedly different effects on the brain.

The amount of power flowing through a system is called a **watt** (1 watt [W] = 1 volt × 1 ampere).

Resistance

Resistance is a measure of how difficult it is to move charges along a conductor. It is measured in **ohms**. If we use the plumbing analogy again, electrical resistance is similar to friction when water flows through a pipe. Longer pipes and pipes with smaller diameter have greater friction, and it is harder to move the water through. A similar situation exists for copper wires and electrical current. Long, thin wires have greater resistance. Resistance also applies to things like toaster ovens and televisions—things that use electricity and slow down the movement of electrons.

Resistance and conductivity are inversely related. Poor conductors have high resistance, whereas good conductors have low resistance. Different materials have different capacity to conduct and resist electricity. Typically, we say that copper is a good conductor with low resistance, whereas rubber is a poor conductor with high resistance. In brain stimulation, the skull is a terrible conductor with high resistance. Different brain tissues such as neurons, spinal fluid, and white matter fiber tracts are generally great conductors with low resistance.

Electroconvulsive therapy (ECT) provides a good example of the relevance of resistance in brain stimulation. The human skull is relatively resistant to the passage of an electrical current. In order to deliver a charge to the brain sufficient enough to induce a seizure, a large-voltage electrical stimulation is applied to the scalp. Much of the current is lost to the skull before it reaches the brain.

Conductance

The conductance of a system is the reciprocal (or opposite) of the resistance. That is, a system with high resistance has low conductance, and vice versa. Conductance is measured in **siemens**.

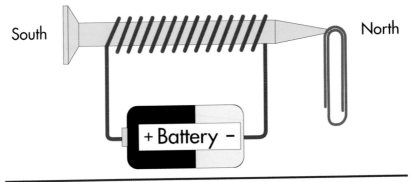

South / North / + Battery –

FIGURE 2–3.   A simple magnet.
When an electrical current flows through a wire, it creates a magnetic field. When the wire is wrapped about a steel nail, the nail becomes magnetized.

Now that we have refreshed the basic concepts and vocabulary of electricity, let's make it even more interesting.

Electromagnetism

Electricity and magnetism are almost interchangeable. When an electric current is passed through a wire, it creates a magnetic field. This is a standard grade-school science project that entails using a battery, some wire, and a nail to make a magnet (Figure 2–3).
    Alternatively, when an object that conducts electricity (meaning something that is willing to give up electrons), such as a copper wire, is passed through a magnetic field, an electrical current is created in the wire (Figure 2–4). The essential point is that the wire must be cutting through the lines of magnetic force. A stationary wire inside a constant nonmoving magnet does not produce an electrical circuit.

Alternating Current

It is the movement of electrons that generates the electromotive force (remember, this pressure or force is called *voltage*). With direct

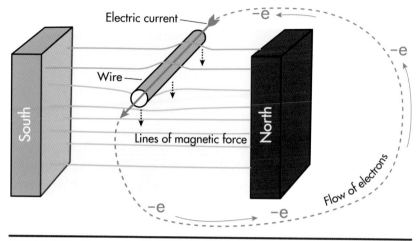

FIGURE 2–4. Inducing an electrical current.
A conductor (in this case a wire) passing through a magnetic field will induce an electrical current and voltage.

current, the electrons all move in the same direction. Electrons can also move back and forth. This is called *alternating current* and is the kind of electricity we get from a household socket. Understanding the mechanics of the electric generators that provide the electricity to our wall sockets is a good way to understand alternating current.

Huge electric generators produce almost all the electrical power people use. A generator does not create energy; rather, it changes mechanical energy into electrical energy. Some form of mechanical energy, such as dammed water, wind, coal, or diesel fuel, must be employed to provide the mechanical energy. The mechanical energy is used to spin a conducting wire inside a magnetic field, which then induces an electrical current (Figure 2–5).

In Figure 2–5 a wire loop is spun clockwise by some mechanical force, such as water rushing out of a dam. In the first frame, the wire "cuts" across the magnetic lines, and an electrical current is induced by the movement of electrons from B to A. When the wire is parallel to the magnetic lines of force (*middle frame*), no lines of force are cut and no electric current is generated. A quarter-turn later, the wire is again cutting through magnetic force, but this time in the opposite direction from the first frame. An electrical current is induced, but the electrons are now moving from A to B. Consequently, as the wire is rapidly turned inside the magnetic field, a current is induced that alternates direction inside the wire.

Figure 2–6 shows the same simple generator but includes a measurement of the voltage (electrical current) induced through one complete turn of the wire loop. When the loop is straight up and down (*a, c,* and *e*), no electrons are moving, and zero voltage is generated. When the loop is cutting across the magnetic force (*b* and *d*), maximum voltage is generated. However, the direction, or *polarity,* of the voltage changes depending on which direction the electrons are flowing. One complete revolution of the loop is called a *cycle.*

War of Currents

The race to corner the market on the distribution of electricity in the 1880s produced a battle between industrial giants. Thomas Edison advocated direct current, while George Westinghouse and Nicola Tesla backed alternating current. Edison, despite all his genius, made the wrong choice. Direct current is less efficient over long distances and would require power plants within a mile of every house or factory. Alternating current can be sent from a few large power plants over long distances at high voltage and then transformed down to a convenient low voltage. However, solar panels transform the sun's energy into direct current, which then is converted into alternating current for practical use. So maybe we *will* have little power plants on each house. Wouldn't Edison be pleased?

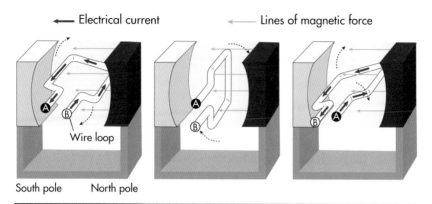

FIGURE 2–5. A simple generator.

A spinning wire loop inside a magnetic field induces an alternating current.

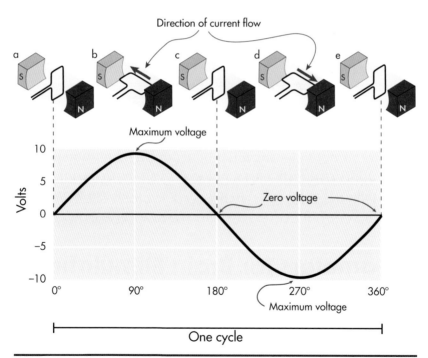

FIGURE 2–6. Alternating current.

Wire spinning inside a magnetic field induces electrical current (voltage) to move in one direction in the first half of the cycle and in the opposite direction in the second half of the cycle.

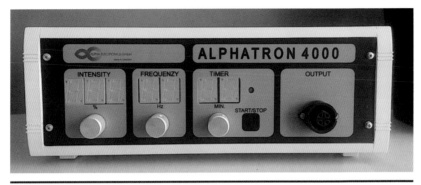

FIGURE 2–7. Alphatron 4000.

Image provided by Johannes Drzyzga, M.Sc.Eng., JSC Technology GmbH/ Hamburg. Used with permission.

The voltage that a generator produces can be increased in several ways:

1. Increase the strength of the magnetic field.
2. Increase the speed at which the wire loop rotates.
3. Increase the number of loops of wire.

One of us (M.S.G.) recently received a most unusual phone call. A local woman died and left him an Alphatron device in her will. Now, we are not endorsing this product and, frankly, cannot vouch for its utility or effectiveness, but look at all the dials on the face of this device (Figure 2–7). What do they do? Well, we address this in the next section.

Parameters for Brain Stimulation

The focal application of electricity to the brain is the focus of this book. The goal with brain stimulation, as with any treatment, is to give enough, but no more than is needed. That is, we strive to produce benefits with minimal side effects. In the following subsections, we review the different parameters that can be modified to adjust the dose of electricity that is given to the brain.

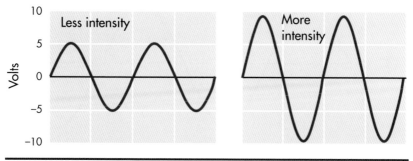

FIGURE 2–8. Intensity.

An electrical stimulation with higher voltage delivers a more intense charge to the brain.

Directionality

Is the electrical signal unidirectional, like direct current, or is it bi-directional, like alternating current? This fundamental difference produces important biological differences.

Intensity

Simply increasing the voltage (pressure) of an electrical stimulation increases the intensity of the charge delivered to the brain (Figure 2–8).

Intensity is important for all the brain stimulation techniques, because there is a minimum amount of electricity needed to interact with a neuron and affect its firing (generate or halt an action potential). This is most easily seen with transcranial magnetic stimulation (TMS) over the thumb region of the motor cortex. Low-intensity stimulation has no effect, but increasingly higher intensity will, at some point (called the *motor threshold*), cause the thumb to twitch.

Frequency

The frequency of an alternating current is the number of cycles per second. For example, power provided by utility companies in the United States is 60 cycles per second, whereas in Europe it is

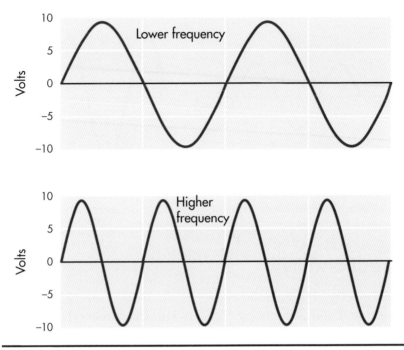

FIGURE 2–9.   Frequency.

The number of cycles per second (hertz) is the frequency of an electrical pulse, shown here with a sine wave alternating current.

50 cycles per second. Cycles per second are called *hertz*, or Hz (Figure 2–9).

Frequency is probably the most important concept for brain stimulation, because different behavioral effects seem to follow frequency-dependent rules. For example, in Chapter 7, "Deep Brain Stimulation and Cortical Stimulation," we review how a parkinsonian tremor only stops with frequencies above 100 Hz, for reasons that are not clear. Similarly, with TMS, low frequencies apparently are inhibitory, whereas high frequencies generally excite tissue.

Pulse Width and Morphology

The pulse width, duration, and even morphology (shape) of the electrical pulse also carry a great deal of importance when applying electricity to the brain. For example, for many years ECT was done with very fat pulse widths. Recently it was discovered that

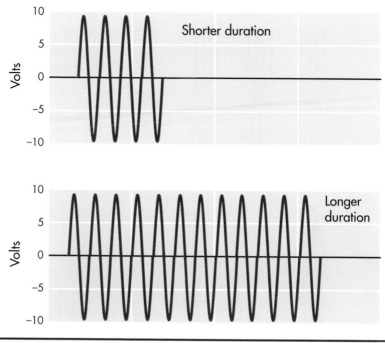

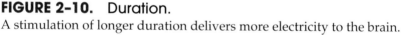

FIGURE 2–10. Duration.

A stimulation of longer duration delivers more electricity to the brain.

most of the electricity in the fat pulse width in ECT was not needed, and in fact this unneeded portion contributed to toxicity (as reviewed in Figure 4–4). Now we have ultra-brief pulse ECT, which is safer and likely just as effective. Fifty years of ECT research can be summarized as the discovery that one can simply change the pulse width to match what a neuron really needs to depolarize and then deliver just that and no more.

Duration

Duration describes the length of the stimulation. It should be self-evident that a stimulation of longer duration as shown in Figure 2–10 delivers more electricity to the brain. However, sometimes it is counterintuitive—a longer duration is not always more effective. This is perhaps one of the harder concepts to understand in the field of brain stimulation, because the brain is dynamic, and different cascading events occur over different time domains, some

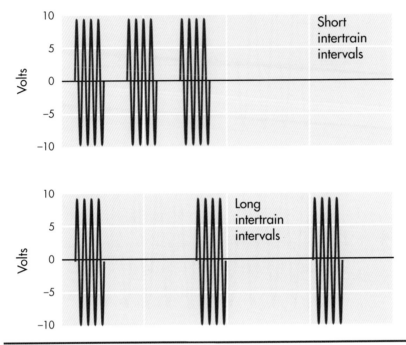

FIGURE 2-11.   Intertrain interval.

Intertrain interval is the time between trains of stimulation.

of which inhibit the effects of the initial stimulation. This duration domain is also one of the most interesting, because it fundamentally is linked to neuronal plasticity.

Intertrain Interval

The intertrain interval describes the length of time between pulses or trains of electrical pulses (Figure 2–11).

The intertrain interval is biologically important because the brain is often responding to the stimulation immediately after a pulse, and a new pulse can have different effects depending on the time between pulses and the amount of time into a train. The brain is thus dynamically responding to the external stimulation and adapting over time. Thus, the length of the train duration is important in the overall effect left from the stimulation. This concept seems to be important with respect to TMS and whether the

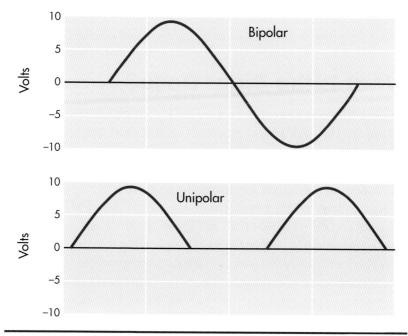

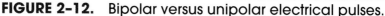

FIGURE 2-12. Bipolar versus unipolar electrical pulses.

brain can return to baseline between trains. With short intertrain intervals, the effects of one train carry into the next train and can build. Thus, continuous short intertrain intervals of TMS can be problematic because they are more likely to cause seizures.

With vagus nerve stimulation a variety of parameters, including the intertrain interval, can be adjusted to improve effectiveness. However, one must be cautious because short intervals can actually damage the nerve (plus it wears out the battery, without any more effectiveness).

Bipolar Versus Unipolar Delivery

We saw earlier that alternating current frequently is bipolar and occurs as a sine wave. As we begin to modify the pulse into rectangular shapes, we can deliver the pulse in either a bipolar or a unipolar manner (Figure 2–12). These two approaches carry different effects. In general, bipolar stimulation is more efficient from the standpoint of delivering electricity. However, in general, unipolar pulses are more efficient in interacting with nerve cells because the actual change in electrical current is what causes depolarization, and the rest of the pulse is not needed to cause neuronal discharge.

What Is the Right Dose?

Pulling all these concepts and terms together, we now have the vocabulary to understand electrical stimulation. We can begin to get a feel for the amount of electricity that the different techniques deliver. To better understand this, it is important to examine how much resting electricity the brain itself creates.

Remember that the human brain itself is an electrical organ, and a highly inefficient one at that. In fact, so much of our daily caloric intake goes into just keeping our brain operating that the question of why this inefficiency was selected for presents an evolutionary puzzle. All day long, even during sleep, the brain is constantly maintaining action potentials and discharging them. The brain represents only 2% of body weight, and yet it receives 15% of the cardiac output, 20% of total body oxygen consumption, and 25% of total body glucose utilization. The energy consumption for the brain to simply survive is 0.1 calories per minute, while this value can be as high as 1.5 calories per minute during complex tasks such as integrating calculus equations.

So, if this is the background electrical activity in the brain, or energy being used, how much are we adding with the different brain stimulation techniques? In general, the answer is very little. Although there is the popular idea that ECT is pumping massive amounts of electricity into the brain, the amount is very small compared with the background resting electrical activity. How small?

As we get more into each of the specific techniques, you will discover that each method differs slightly. For example, those techniques that are intermittent (such as ECT or TMS) use less electricity than those that are constantly on (such as deep brain stimulation). We need a few more terms to best discuss this. Remember that current is the flow of electrons. If we describe the flow of electrons in a specific space or bit of tissue, that is called the **current density**, measured in *joules*. In the next chapter we see that when we pass electricity through a nerve cell, the current density turns into a

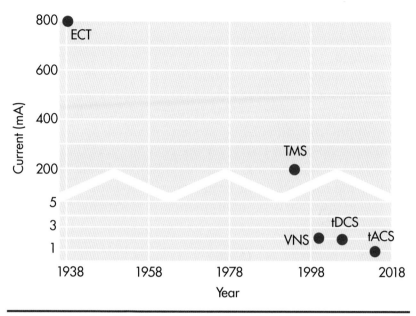

FIGURE 2–13. Reduced need for electrical dose in brain stimulation therapies.

The dose of current given for each device when first used as a therapy on human subjects.

charge density, which builds up on a neuronal membrane. We can then calculate the specific absorption of energy per pulse—or considered over time, the **specific absorption rate** (SAR). The SAR is an important concept for many medical devices, such as ultrasounds and magnetic resonance imaging (MRI) scans, that deposit energy into the body or brain. There are strict guidelines for the SAR limits on modern MRI scanners, for instance.

Yet how much energy do the devices deposit, compared with normal brain activity? Well, the SAR of a typical TMS pulse at 1 Hz is about 2 mW/kg, while the resting brain metabolic rate is 13 W/kg. If the average adult brain weighs 1,300 g, or 1.3 kg, then TMS at 1 Hz is adding 0.002/17 W/kg, or 0.012% more energy. The other techniques are also in this ballpark. Even the energy deposited with ECT, which is perceived as delivering large amounts of energy, is small compared to the background electrical energy of the brain. In ECT, the typical current is 800 milliamps, delivered for 1–6 seconds. If most people respond in 10 treatments, the total time of exposure is 10–60 seconds, and around 8,000 milliamps delivered over a full treatment course. This is a small amount of energy indeed.

In one sense, the different brain stimulation methods have become more focal and more efficient at interacting with the brain while delivering less electricity. Figure 2–13 shows how the different approaches differ by the amount of current applied during a pulse, or dose, and how over the past 80 years the field has tended to use less and less. And this is how it should be. If electricity is the currency of the brain, we need to learn how to actually talk to the brain with small amounts of electricity, rather than SHOUTING.

References

George MS, Belmaker RH: Transcranial Magnetic Stimulation in Clinical Psychiatry. Washington, DC, American Psychiatric Publishing, 2007

Rosenberg P, Middleton R: Audel Practical Electricity, 5th Edition. New York, Wiley, 2004

CHAPTER 3

Electrical Brain

Getting Started

The previous two chapters focused on the general principles of electricity in wires and circuits. However, the really important issue for brain stimulation is how electricity works within biological systems—nerves and cells. Here we show how the principles from Chapters 1 and 2 are modified to actually work within neurons.

Intracellular Charge

All living cells possess an electrical charge, with the inside of the cell more negatively charged than the outside (Rosenzweig et al. 2005). The resting membrane potential is approximately –50 to –80 milli-

volts (mV) in a nerve cell. Nerve cells use this property to communicate with one another.

This negative charge inside a cell is maintained through three
general mechanisms:

1. Electrostatic pressure
2. Concentration gradient
3. Sodium-potassium pump

Cells contain large negatively charged molecules (e.g., proteins, DNA) that are trapped inside a cell and cannot cross the cell
membrane. These large molecules attract positively charged ions
such as sodium and potassium. However, the cell membrane is
selectively permeable to these ions. Potassium can easily pass
through ion channels, but other ions such as sodium and chloride
cannot.

The electrostatic pressure on the potassium is relatively strong
and draws a disproportionate amount of the potassium ions into
the cell. As the ions accumulate inside the cell, there is increasing
concentration pressure pulling the potassium back out of the cell.
These competing and opposing forces reach an equilibrium in
which potassium is predominantly intracellular (Figure 3–1). The
mnemonic that many people use is KIN, for potassium (K) IN-
side the cell. This results in a resting membrane potential of about
–65 mV.

Sodium-Potassium Pump

The positively charged sodium ions, much like 2-year-old children, are not entirely cooperative. They keep going where they
shouldn't—in this case, into the cell. Left unchecked, the sodium
would eventually neutralize the negative electrostatic charge inside the cell. Consequently, cells have developed a mechanism to
continually return sodium ions to the extracellular space. The sodium-potassium pump schematically drawn in Figure 3–2 swaps
intracellular sodium ions for extracellular potassium ions. The
end result is high concentration gradients across the cell wall for
potassium and sodium. This becomes important for the rapid propagation of the action potential.

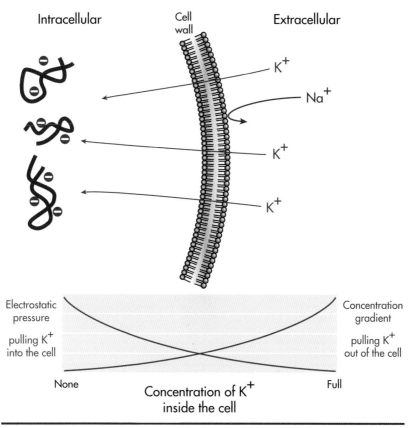

FIGURE 3–1. The electrostatic/concentration tug of war.
The large, negatively charged molecules inside the cell pull on the positively charged potassium ions. As the concentration of potassium increases inside the cell, the concentration gradient pulls the ions out.

Nerve Cell Structures

A brief review of nerve cell structures is necessary before proceeding further. Nerve cells can be divided into three zones: input, conduction, and output (Figure 3–3). The dendrites are the input zone of the cell, or what some call the "ears" of the neuron. They are covered with synaptic terminals that can receive signals from other neurons. If the electrical charge reaches the threshold at the axon hillock, then an impulse, or *action potential*, is sent down the axon. That signal is passed on to other neurons or end organs through the synaptic terminals at the distal end of the nerve.

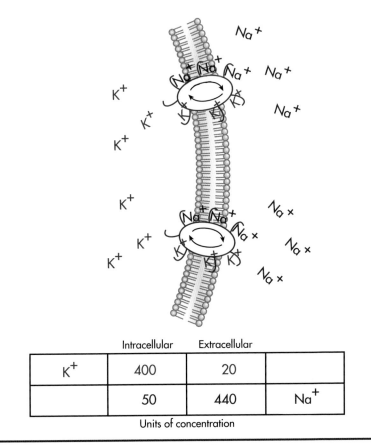

	Intracellular	Extracellular	
K^+	400	20	
	50	440	Na^+

Units of concentration

FIGURE 3-2. The sodium-potassium pump.

The sodium-potassium pump swaps sodium and potassium ions to maintain a high concentration gradient across the cell wall.

Generating an Action Potential

Dendrites receive as many as 100,000 inputs from other nerve cells. How does the nerve cell "decide" if it should respond and fire its own impulse? The decision to fire an impulse is determined by the membrane potential at the axon hillock. The membrane potential is altered by input to the dendrites from other neurons. Some inputs depolarize the neuron and make it more likely to fire an action potential, while other inputs hyperpolarize the neu-

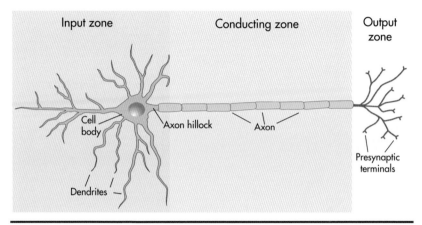

FIGURE 3-3. Nerve cell structures.

Nerve cells can be conceptualized as having an input zone (dendrites), a conducting zone (axon), and an output zone (synapses formed with neurons or glands).

ron and make it less likely to fire. The "decision" to fire is thus a mathematical vote of all of the competing inputs to the cell, some of which push to depolarize and fire whereas others reduce the likelihood of firing. The currency of the brain is electricity, and each of the billions of cells in the brain is constantly "deciding" whether or not to pass the message on. The sum total of many nerves firing produces thoughts, feeling, movement, and decisions. Fascinating, really.

Excitatory or Inhibitory

Excitatory neurons (predominantly glutamate neurons) are depolarizing neurons. An influx of positively charged sodium ions from these neurons results in a more positive membrane potential that is more likely to fire an action potential. Inhibitory neurons (predominantly γ-aminobutyric acid [GABA] neurons) are hyperpolarizing neurons. An influx of negatively charged chloride ions from these neurons results in a more negative membrane potential that is less likely to fire. In other words, the movement of charged ions into the nerve cell at the synapses alters the electrical potential of the cell. This process is illustrated in Figure 3–4.

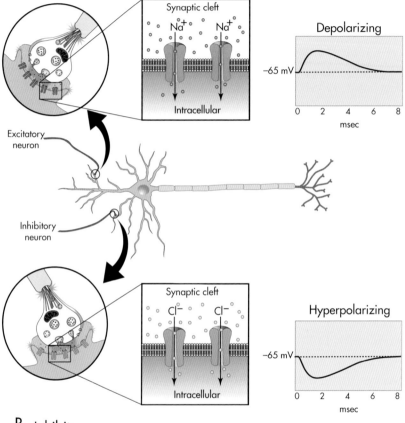

A Excitatory

Synaptic cleft

Na^+ Na^+

Depolarizing

−65 mV

Intracellular

0   2   4   6   8
msec

Excitatory neuron

Inhibitory neuron

Synaptic cleft

Cl^- Cl^-

Hyperpolarizing

−65 mV

Intracellular

0   2   4   6   8
msec

B Inhibitory

FIGURE 3–4. Excitatory and inhibitory inputs.

Input from an excitatory neuron **(A)** depolarizes the receiving neuron.
Input from an inhibitory neuron **(B)** hyperpolarizes the receiving neuron.

Axon Hillock

The response of the neuron depends on the electrical charge at the
axon hillock (Purves et al. 2004). This is where the "decision" is
made. The neuron will fire and send an action potential down the
axon if the membrane potential reaches the threshold at the axon
hillock. The membrane potential at the axon hillock is a summation

of the depolarizing and hyperpolarizing signals received by the dendrites. Figure 3–5 shows how different input from other neurons alters the membrane potential at the axon hillock, which in turn determines whether the neuron fires and an action potential is sent down the axon.

Action Potential

The "all or none" aspect of the action potential is one of the important features of the signal. Once the threshold is reached at the axon hillock, the neuron sends a large, uniform electric signal down its own axon. The electric charge results from the large and rapid influx of positively charged sodium ions into the negatively charged intracellular space. The ability to pass the signal down the axon with no diminution in its strength allows the signal to travel great distances, for example, the length of the spinal cord of a whale.

A few words about myelin. The oligodendrocytes (one of the glial cells—nonneuronal cells in the brain) wrap myelin around the axons, which increases the speed of electrical transmissions. Most myelin is wrapped after birth and correlates with the maturing of the brain. Conversely, demyelinating diseases, such as multiple sclerosis, slow transmission of electrical signaling, which impairs brain function.

Chemical Signal

Ultimately, the action potential arrives at the terminal end of the neuron (see Figure 1–1). Here the electrical signal induces an influx of calcium, which in turn results in fusing of the neurotransmitter-filled vesicles with the synaptic cell wall. The neurotransmitters are dumped into the synaptic cleft and, if sufficient, stimulate the next neuron or end organ.

So, repeat this basic sequence 100 billion times (the number of neurons), and some of these firing many times per minute, and you have the summed electrical activity of the brain. Remember from the last chapter that this consumes a little less than 0.1 calorie per minute (40–50 calories per hour, or 900–1,200 calories per day) just to keep all those action potentials charged and to recharge the axon hillock after sending off an action potential. This sym-

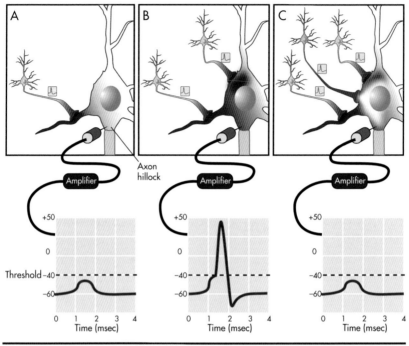

FIGURE 3–5. Reaching the threshold.

Input from one excitatory neuron **(A)** does not increase the membrane potential enough to reach the threshold. Input from two excitatory neurons **(B)** pushes the membrane potential at the axon hillock over the threshold, and an action potential is fired. The additional input of an inhibitory neuron **(C)** hyperpolarizes the neuron, and the membrane potential again does not reach the threshold.

phony of discharges becomes unbelievably complex, but it all starts from these basic building blocks. The brain stimulation techniques by and large modify this basic mechanism in selected brain regions or circuits by introducing focal electrical stimulation or by modulating these key variables involved in electrical flow.

Clinical Relevance

Electroencephalography

As early as 1875, electrical activity had been recorded from the exposed cerebral cortex of a monkey (Bear et al. 2006). However, it was Hans Berger, a German psychiatrist, who in 1929 first recorded electroencephalographic (EEG) scalp tracings from awake humans. Berger became interested in "brain waves" after he had been thrown from a horse in a forest far from home. At precisely the time of his injury his sister, in a distant town, suddenly sensed he was in danger and demanded that he be contacted. Berger always wondered how this had happened and many years later started looking for signals coming out of the brain. Berger went on to show that different states of the brain produced different EEG rhythms. The EEG remains a useful tool for understanding epilepsy and sleep.

Extrasensory Perception

While there are numerous anecdotal stories of extrasensory perception (ESP), it is not likely that Berger's electroencephalographic signals contacted his sister about his dangerous predicament. Systematic scientific studies of ESP have failed to demonstrate mental telepathy between two people. However, it remains possible (and likely probable) that the brain gives off signals that have yet to be discovered.

EEG recordings are generally made through two dozen electrodes fixed to the scalp in predetermined locations. The electrodes are connected to amplifiers and recording devices. Small voltage changes are measured between pairs of electrodes. Usually the voltage fluctuations are only a few tens of microvolts in amplitude.

The EEG measures a summation of electrical activity from a large number of neurons beneath the electrode. Research with animals has determined that most of the electrical activity being recorded is coming from synaptic activity on the dendrites of the large pyramidal neurons. Figure 3–6 shows a schematic diagram of how this is happening. Signals from afferent neurons release the neurotransmitter at the synapse. The movement of positive

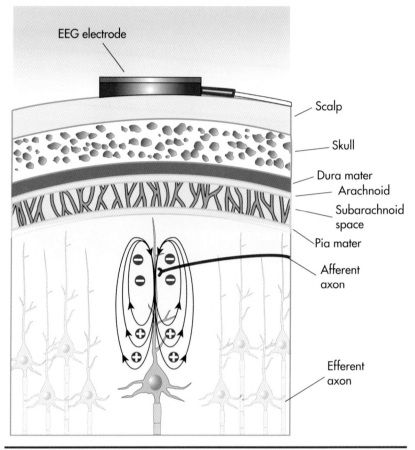

FIGURE 3–6. Synaptic activity produces a slight electrical charge.

When thousands of other cells contribute their small voltage, a signal becomes strong enough to be detected by the electroencephalographic electrode at the scalp.

Source.   Adapted from Bear et al. 2006.

ions into the pyramidal neuron leaves a slightly negative charge in the extracellular fluid. As the current spreads and escapes out of the deeper parts of the neuron, those extracellular sites become slightly positive.

EEG recordings are measuring the summation of activity from thousands of neurons. If the activity is out of synch or irregular, then the EEG summation will have a high frequency and small am-

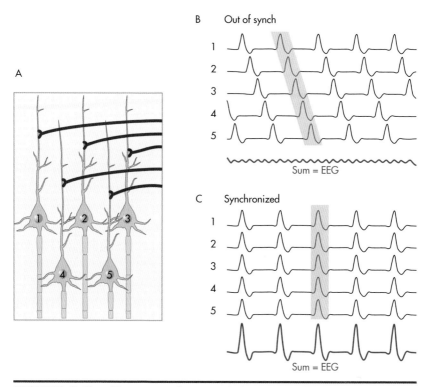

FIGURE 3–7. How synchrony determines EEG frequency.

Activity from five neurons is being recorded **(A)**. When the signals are out of synch and irregular, the summation (*shown in red*) will record high-frequency, low-amplitude EEG waves **(B)**. Synchronized signals produce low-frequency, high-amplitude EEG recordings **(C)**.

plitude. On the other hand, if the activity is synchronized, then the EEG summation will be low-frequency, high-amplitude waves. Figure 3–7 gives an example of this summation. In other words, the characteristics of the EEG waves are reflecting the synchrony of the neurons, not some measure of their activity.

As we discussed in the previous chapter, electricity and magnetic fields are interchangeable, and whenever electrical current flows, there is a magnetic field induced around the wire (or axon). Magnetoencephalography (MEG) is a functional imaging technology that measures brain activity by recording the magnetic fields produced by electrical currents in the brain. Although very expensive and only used in research as this time, MEG is the magnetic equivalent of electroencephalography, recording the tiny magnetic field changes caused by synchronous neuronal firing. MEG has the advantage of less distortion from skull and scalp. MEG also offers the ability to follow brain activity, much as with functional magnetic resonance imaging (fMRI), but about 10 times faster.

One of the more interesting ideas within the field of brain stimulation involves modifying the stimulation based on the EEG data or some other physiological reading—sort of the brain equivalent of dosing insulin based on real-time blood sugar levels. This is called "closed loop" stimulation, where the stimulation is constantly modified by or triggered from some signal coming out of the subject. In deep brain stimulation, this has been called *responsive stimulation therapy* and has been pioneered largely by one company, NeuroPace, for treating epilepsy. The same or a similar idea of tailoring the stimulation based on the EEG or some other biomarker is being investigated with the other brain stimulation techniques.

It gets even a bit more complicated, or interesting, depending on your perspective. Remember that each neuron has a resting potential, and when the neuron is fired and sends an action potential, electricity begins flowing through the axon, which in turn generates a magnetic field around it. If we place neurons in a petri dish, they will sometimes grow into organized bundles. Then, as one neuron fires, producing changes in magnetic fields, it influences the neighboring neurons. Over time, these cells begin firing in synchrony, producing their own form of synchronous EEG. Thus, the organized cells begin acting as a unit, producing a common electromagnetic field. We find this exciting because it shows you can then influence the electromagnetic field through precise rhythmic but very weak electromagnetic stimulation and thus change the firing patterns of the whole dish ("presto chango"). This concept is behind the new areas of *transcranial alternating current stimulation*, which we discuss later in the book.

Sleep

The frequency and amplitude of the EEG best reflect the state of alertness of the individual (Higgins and George 2019). EEG recordings from awake and asleep individuals show the changes in EEG rhythms. Figure 3–8 shows examples of different rhythms and

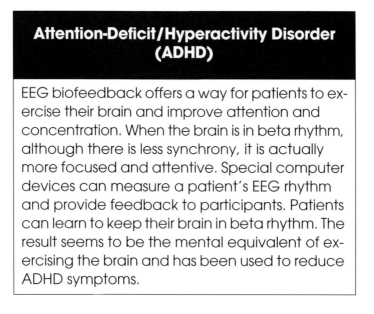

Rhythm	Mental state	Example	Frequency
Beta	active attention		14–16 Hz
Alpha	quiet awake		8–13 Hz
Theta	drowsy / light sleep		4–7 Hz
Delta	deep sleep		<4 Hz

FIGURE 3–8. EEG rhythms.

The four basic EEG rhythms of the brain during sleep and awake states.

the usual mental state associated with each. Higher-frequency rhythms such as beta rhythm are found when individuals are alert and focused. Slower waveforms such as theta and delta are found during sleep. Signals from the thalamus seem to be driving the synchronization of the cortical neurons during sleep. However, it remains unclear why this synchronization is an important aspect of the sleeping brain.

Attention-Deficit/Hyperactivity Disorder (ADHD)

EEG biofeedback offers a way for patients to exercise their brain and improve attention and concentration. When the brain is in beta rhythm, although there is less synchrony, it is actually more focused and attentive. Special computer devices can measure a patient's EEG rhythm and provide feedback to participants. Patients can learn to keep their brain in beta rhythm. The result seems to be the mental equivalent of exercising the brain and has been used to reduce ADHD symptoms.

Seizures

A *seizure* is the rhythmic firing of large groups of neurons. It is the most extreme form of synchronous brain activity. Inducing a seizure for therapeutic benefits becomes the focus of treatment discussed in Chapter 4, "Electroconvulsive Therapy." However, spontaneous seizures are a sign of a disorder. Much of the focus with new-onset seizures is directed toward finding the cause of the problem: infection, electrolyte imbalance, medications, alcohol, and so on.

Summary to This Point

We have thus far reviewed the basics of electricity and circuits, introduced many basic concepts and terms, and discussed how neurons use chemical gradients to propagate electrical information. With this information in hand, we can now begin discussing the brain stimulation technologies, where we use some form of focal electrical or magnetic energy to modify brain activity.

References

Bear MF, Connors BW, Paradiso MA: Neuroscience: Exploring the Brain. Baltimore, MD, Lippincott Williams & Wilkins, 2006

Higgins ES, George MS: The Neuroscience of Clinical Psychiatry: The Pathophysiology of Behavior and Mental Illness, 3rd Edition. Philadelphia, PA, Wolters Kluwer/Lippincott, Williams & Wilkins, 2019

Purves D, Augustine GJ, Fitzpatrick D, et al: Neuroscience, 3rd Edition. Sunderland, MA, Sinauer, 2004

Rosenzweig MR, Breedlove SM, Watson NV: Biological Psychology, 4th Edition. Sunderland, MA, Sinauer, 2005

CHAPTER 4

Electroconvulsive Therapy

Introduction and History

Eighty years ago as we write this text, the Italian physician Ugo Cerletti was the first clinician to utilize electroconvulsive therapy (ECT) as a treatment for a psychiatric patient (Shorter 2004). The year was 1938. The idea to induce a seizure with an electrical pulse as a therapeutic intervention for a psychiatric disorder was not entirely out of the blue. "Physical therapies," such as malarial-fever treatment for neurosyphilis, were emerging as effective treatments for psychiatric illnesses. Chemically induced convulsive therapies had been introduced in 1934.

Chemically induced seizures involved the intramuscular administration of camphor, and later pentylenetetrazol, to elicit a therapeutic seizure (Prudic 2005). The procedure had some success, which was remarkable during that time, when few treatment options were available. In one report, approximately 50% of the patients had some degree of reduction of their psychotic symptoms after an intervention. Unfortunately, chemically induced seizures were painful and could be difficult to control. Some lasted significantly longer than desired. Flurothyl gas was also used to induce convulsive seizures, but the gas sometimes leaked and affected caregivers! The introduction of an electrically stimulated convulsion by Cerletti and his assistant Bini introduced a much-improved method to induce a therapeutic seizure. They could precisely time when the seizure might occur, rather than waiting for medications to slowly work.

Cerletti had theorized that electricity might provide a safer method of inducing convulsions. Working first with dogs and then with pigs, Cerletti established a safe mechanism to evoke a seizure without harming the animal. The story of the first person to receive ECT represents one of the landmark interventions of psychiatry (Cerletti 1950).

The patient was a 39-year-old former engineer who was found wandering the Italian streets in a delusional state. He was unable to speak coherently and appeared to have no family. He was diagnosed with schizophrenia; he failed to improve, and his prognosis was poor. By modern standards, such a patient would not be able to consent to an untested intervention. However, at that time he was considered an ideal candidate and was prepped for the procedure.

The first electrical stimulation administered, unfortunately, did not induce a seizure. At the prospect of receiving a second stimulation the otherwise uncommunicative patient exclaimed, "Not a *second*. Deadly!" Cerletti was not to be deterred. The voltage and duration were increased and a second jolt given. This time the patient had a true seizure and actually stopped breathing for almost a minute. Cerletti later wrote what happened next: "The patient sat up of his own accord, looked about him calmly with a vague smile, as though asking what was expected of him. I asked him:

'What has been happening to you?' He answered, with no more gibberish: 'I don't know; perhaps I have been asleep'" (Cerletti 1950, p. 91).

The patient received 10 more ECT sessions in the following weeks and had a remarkable recovery. Within 2 months, he was reunited with his wife and eventually resumed his job. A year later he was still working and living at home. Cerletti established with cases like this that ECT was effective and reasonably safe.

The psychiatric community quickly embraced ECT. In 1940, ECT was demonstrated at the annual meeting of the American Psychiatric Association (Shorter 2004). The following year a group in Boston (where else?) published a handbook on ECT. Refinements in the technique further enhanced the acceptance of ECT. The addition of succinylcholine and anesthesia reduced problems associated with the procedure, such as fractures incurred during the muscular contractions induced by the seizure. By 1959, which may have been the high-water mark for the procedure, ECT was the "treatment of choice" for major depression and bipolar disorder (Shorter 1997). However, that was soon to change.

Chlorpromazine (Thorazine), introduced in 1954, and imipramine (Tofranil), in 1958, were the first effective antipsychotic and antidepressant medications (Shorter 1997). Now there were three options for patients: psychotherapy, medications, and brain stimulation. Utilization of ECT dropped dramatically, not only because of the availability of pharmacological interventions but also because of a sociocultural rejection of ECT (Shorter 2004).

Overutilization is a common phenomenon in mental health treatment, and ECT was no exception. Unfortunately, some patients felt abused; the procedure looks barbaric when used without anesthesia, and it drew the ire of the antipsychiatrist movement. The novel (1962), and later movie (1975), *One Flew Over the Cuckoo's Nest* had a devastating effect on the public perception of ECT. State legislators started passing laws to restrict the use of ECT.

Fortunately, since the mid-1980s the tide has begun to turn (Dukakis and Tye 2006). There has been a resurgence of interest in ECT (along with other brain stimulation therapies). Training programs resumed teaching the procedure, and increasing numbers of patients are benefiting from the treatment. In fact, despite

80 years of advancements in the field, no treatment is more effective for depression than ECT. Although indicated for a range of disorders, ECT is typically reserved for severely depressed, manic, or catatonic patients who fail to respond to other treatments or those who have life-threatening conditions in need of emergent resolution.

How Is It Done?

If we think of ECT as a meal, the essential ingredient is the seizure. Inducing a seizure is *necessary* for therapeutic benefits (although not every seizure is therapeutic). In a classic study in 1960, Cronholm and Ottosson established that it was the seizure activity that produced the therapeutic response with ECT and not just the electrical activity. They did this by randomly administering an anticonvulsant (lidocaine) to some of the patients prior to ECT. Those who received the lidocaine displayed less seizure activity, required more electrical stimulation, and did not respond as well. Cronholm and Ottosson concluded, in regard to ECT, that the seizure is necessary but not sufficient to produce the therapeutic effect.

Modern ECT, at least in the United States and other industrialized nations, is administered with brief anesthesia, muscle relaxants, and supplemental oxygen. In some third-world countries, such amenities are not provided. Figure 4–1 shows the general components of ECT. The ECT device takes power from an external source and delivers a brief impulse through the paddles or pads to the patient's scalp. The electrical stimulation must be sufficient to induce a seizure.

Dosing

The general principles of brain stimulation parameters (frequency, intensity, and duration) apply to ECT. Sufficient stimulation is needed to produce a seizure, but any stimulation above the threshold only increases side effects. The scalp and particularly the skull impede the flow of electricity to the brain—called *resistance*. Patients have varying amounts of resistance to the electrical charge: as much as 50-fold (Prudic 2005). A particular dose for one patient

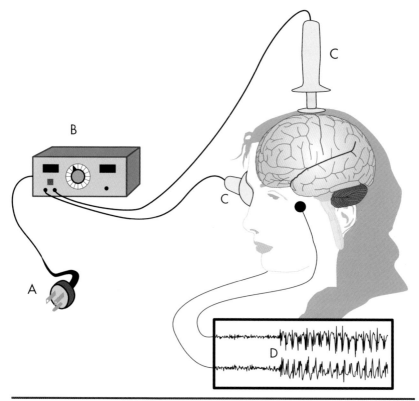

FIGURE 4-1. The ECT apparatus.

With modern ECT, electricity (alternating current) from the wall **(A)** is then stored and released through the ECT device **(B)**. The electrical pulse from the device is commonly a brief pulse (milliseconds). More recent work with ultrabrief pulse has reduced the width of this signal even further, to where it now approaches *chronaxie*, which is the minimum needed to cause an action potential in a nerve. The current is passed through electrodes on the scalp **(C)**, inducing a seizure. Commonly, electroencephalographs and electromyographs (from a nonparalyzed part of the body, typically the foot) are recorded to document the seizure **(D)**.

may be too much or insufficient for another. The goal is to find the "just-right" dose for each patient—the smallest dose possible to produce a seizure.

Many ECT practitioners use published scales or algorithms based on age and sex in order to estimate the appropriate dose.

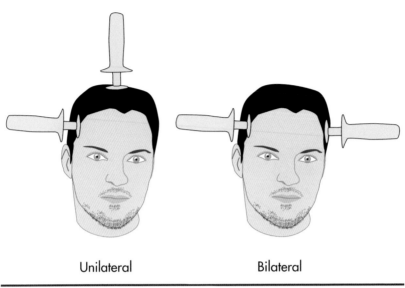

Unilateral   Bilateral

FIGURE 4-2.   Unilateral and bilateral electrode placement for ECT.

Others use a method called *dose titration*. Electricity is delivered in ever increasing amounts until a seizure occurs, in essence finding the seizure threshold. In the subsequent sessions the dose is based on this initial amount, for example, six or nine times the seizure threshold. Typically, the seizure threshold also rises over the several weeks of the ECT course, as the brain responds to the seizure and attempts to prevent future ones. Some even speculate that the antidepressant effects of ECT may be linked to this progressive increase in seizure threshold, although this view is not widely accepted.

Electrode Placement

The placement of the electrodes on the head has a significant effect on both the outcome and side effects. The two most commonly used positions are *bilateral* and *right unilateral* as shown in Figure 4–2. Until 10 years ago, bilateral was more widely used presumably because of increased efficacy. However, bilateral ECT is also associated with greater cognitive side effects. Sackeim et al. (2000)

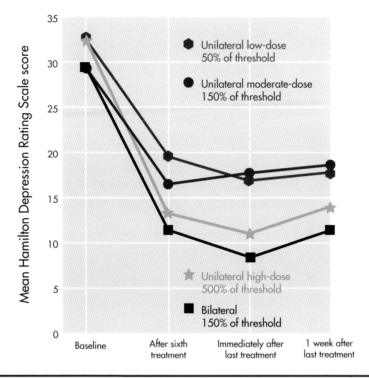

FIGURE 4–3. Electrode placement and depression response.

Mean reduction in Hamilton Depression Rating Scale for different doses of unilateral ECT compared with bilateral ECT.

Source. Adapted from Sackeim et al. 2000.

established that unilateral ECT has fewer side effects even though it requires a larger pulse of electricity to induce a seizure.

The Sackeim et al. (2000) study has had a big impact on the practice of ECT. In that study, 80 depressed patients were randomly assigned to receive unilateral ECT with electrical stimulation at 50%, 150%, or 500% above the seizure threshold or bilateral ECT at 150% of the seizure threshold. Figure 4–3 shows the reductions in mean Hamilton Depression Rating Scale scores: high-dose unilateral ECT and bilateral ECT were equally effective. Two measures of cognitive function are shown in Tables 4–1 and 4–2. Table 4–1 shows the time to recover in minutes. In this case, *recovery* is defined as the return of orientation. Table 4–2 shows

TABLE 4–1.   Time to recover orientation, in minutes, from four different versions of ECT

Low-dose unilateral	Moderate-dose unilateral	High-dose unilateral	Bilateral
19	17	31	46

TABLE 4–2.   Retrograde amnesia for sets of words, shapes, and expressive faces memorized prior to the procedure

Low-dose unilateral	Moderate-dose unilateral	High-dose unilateral	Bilateral
4	0	–2	–17

Note.   A higher number represents less retrograde amnesia.

the results of a test of memory conducted 5 minutes after the patients recovered orientation. The study authors concluded, "Right unilateral ECT at high dosage is as effective as a robust form of bilateral ECT, but produces less severe and persistent cognitive effects" (Sackeim et al. 2000, p. 425).

Waveform

The ECT machine determines the shape of the electrical signal—called the *waveform*. Figure 4–4 shows three commonly used waveforms. The *sine wave* is the older, original waveform. This alternating current waveform is what emerges from a wall socket. The *brief pulse waveform* has the advantage of inducing a seizure with less electrical stimulation. Note the area under the curves and the milliseconds of phase duration are smaller for the brief pulse.

The old sine waveform produces excess electrical stimulation without added benefits. Once the nerve cell has fired, it enters a refractory period during which additional electrical energy is unwar-

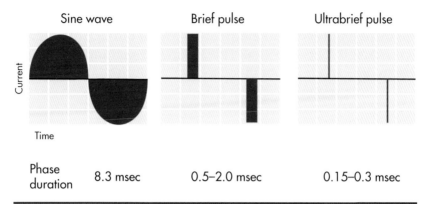

FIGURE 4–4. ECT waveforms.

An example of one cycle for three different waveforms from different ECT machines. Note that historically the sine wave was used in the middle of the twentieth century, followed by the brief pulse in the 1980s, and within the past few years, the ultrabrief pulse.

ranted and probably increases side effects (more on this later). In the past 15 years, scientists have begun using what is called *ultrabrief pulses*. Here the pulses are on the order of milliseconds and are much more "physiological" in terms of what is minimally needed to cause depolarization. In the 10 years since the first edition of this book, most ECT practitioners have switched to using ECT machines that produce an ultrabrief waveform. Right unilateral ultrabrief ECT has largely equal efficacy to bilateral ECT, and reduced cognitive side effects, although it may take a few more treatments with right unilateral ultrabrief ECT to get the same clinical effect (Sackeim et al. 2008). Unfortunately, some older machines remain in use.

Location

You would intuitively think that one grand mal seizure is as good as the next when it comes to alleviating depression, but it turns out not all seizures are equally beneficial. In many cases, for ECT to work, much more electricity than is needed must be given in order to initiate a seizure. A seizure alone is not sufficient. The important variables seem to be both where the seizure starts and the amount of current passed through the tissue. Whatever "secret sauce" is created with ECT (the "secret sauce" that improves mood), it is only created if the seizure originates in beneficial areas of the brain and more electricity is passed through this region. For example, Sackeim et al. (1993) showed that unilateral ECT electrodes can induce a full tonic-clonic seizure but have a minimal antidepressant effect if only just enough to induce a seizure is given. So, a seizure is necessary but not sufficient. Furthermore, a seizure alone does not produce the antidepressant effects of ECT. The seizure must originate in specific regions and be powerful enough to generate the "secret sauce."

Which region of the brain is the optimum location to start a seizure? The general consensus is that the frontal lobes are ideal. However, because the skull acts as a resistor, it is hard to focus exactly where an ECT seizure is induced. Better placement of the electrodes can help direct the pulse toward the frontal lobes and away from the temporal lobes (involved in memory), but it is not perfect. The other problem is that brain regions vary in their tendency to seize. The regions of the brain with the lowest seizure threshold (and thus most likely to start seizing first) are the medial temporal lobe structures (including the hippocampus) and the motor cortex. The frontal lobes are more stubborn.

The astute readers among you may have noticed a conundrum. If a seizure in specific areas is needed for the therapeutic effects of ECT, how did generalized chemical convulsions treat depression? We do not know for sure, but remember that even chemically induced seizures have to start in some specific brain region first. Thus, it may be that the medications or inhalational gases used prior to the development of ECT machines started seizures in the very regions that needed a boost.

Focal Seizures

The holy grail of ECT is to induce a focal seizure in the frontal lobes. A focal seizure, if done correctly, would not generalize to the rest of the brain. If such a procedure were possible, patients would not lose consciousness and would not have disrupted memory because the hippocampus would not be affected. The induced seizure would be similar to an absence seizure (petit mal seizure). Theoretically, if we never had a full convulsion involving the whole body, we could skip the muscle relaxants and send the anesthesiologists home.

One method attempting to do this is called *magnetic seizure therapy* (MST; Sackeim 1994). With this therapy, a powerful transcranial magnetic stimulation (TMS) device (see Chapter 6) is used to create a focal seizure. MST has been done in humans, with several small clinical trials completed. The data so far show that subjects wake up quicker after an MST seizure than they do after an ECT seizure. A recent study found that MST was equivalent to conventional ECT, but both approaches had surprisingly low response rates, raising questions about the patients or overall design of this study (Fitzgerald et al. 2018). MST is an active area of research as a new way to deliver a novel form of seizure therapy.

Another technique to produce a more focal seizure is called *focal electrically applied seizure therapy* (or FEAST—which we love because it perpetuates our theme of cooking-up the perfect meal in the brain). FEAST works by making the electrical stimulus unidirectional—more like direct current. Through use of a small electrode for stimulation and a large reference electrode, current is concentrated under the smaller stimulating electrode placed over the right orbitofrontal cortex, just above the right eyebrow. By delivering this unidirectional current in a pulsatile way, one might induce enough charge to cause a focal seizure just in the right prefrontal lobe. This has been done in primates and in some open-label trials with humans (Nahas et al. 2013; Sahlem et al. 2016; Spellman et al. 2009). These small-sample open-label studies showed that FEAST can preferentially stimulate the frontal lobes, achieve efficacy roughly similar to that of ECT, and result in less memory impairment than that seen with even the briefest pulse form of ECT. Figure 4–5 shows the electrical distribution for right unilateral ultrabrief ECT and FEAST. Note how the electricity collects around the temporal lobes with ECT but stays in the frontal lobes with FEAST.

The absence of temporal lobe involvement with FEAST appears to reduce cognitive side effects compared with ECT. For example, time to recover orientation as shown in Table 4–1 is typically 19 minutes for low-dose unilateral, 17 minutes for moderate-dose unilateral, and 46 for bilateral ECT. Measurements of autobiographical memory (a topic addressed later in Figure 4–7) show less impair-

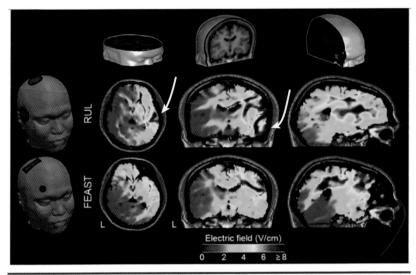

FIGURE 4–5.   Right unilateral ultrabrief ECT compared with focal electrically applied seizure therapy (FEAST) showing electric field distribution.

The *white arrows* show the electrical signal extending into the temporal lobes with the ECT. The *red arrow* points to the majority of the electrical signal pooling in the frontal cortex with FEAST.

Source.   Reprinted with permission from Spellman T, Peterchev AV, Lisanby SH: "Focal Electrically Administered Seizure Therapy: A Novel Form of ECT Illustrates the Roles of Current Directionality, Polarity, and Electrode Configuration in Seizure Induction." *Neuropsychopharmacology* 34(8):2002–2010, 2009. Copyright 2009, American College of Neuropsychopharmacology. Used with permission.

ment with FEAST than with ECT. Large randomized studies are needed (and have been proposed) to test the effectiveness and adverse events for the best modern forms of ECT and FEAST.

Anesthesia

One of the worst features of ECT was the use of the procedure without sedation or paralyzing the body. Although the patient rarely remembered the ECT seizure because of the amnestic side effects of the treatment and seizure, the process looked primitive with the patient thrashing about and the staff holding limbs. Not infrequently, it resulted in orthopedic problems. Fortunately, the development and use of anesthesia during the ECT session has changed all that. Typically, patients are given a muscle relaxer and a general anesthetic. The muscle relaxer, usually succinylcholine, paralyzes the body and stops the actual motor convulsions, preventing bruising and fractures. A blood pressure cuff is usually inflated around the ankle, which prevents the succinylcholine from entering the foot. The nerve impulses are not blocked, and the psychiatrist is able to observe the convulsions from the seizure in the nonparalyzed foot.

With regard to general anesthetics, most hospitals in the United States now use a short-acting barbiturate (methohexital [Brevital] or propofol). Propofol paradoxically raises the seizure threshold, making it harder to induce a seizure. An interesting new trend is to use ketamine. Ketamine, without ECT, has been reported to have antidepressant effects, so the combination of ECT and ketamine would seem to be a reasonable choice. Many clinicians complain, however, that the recovery time is slower from ketamine than from propofol, and ketamine sometimes induces unusual fear or psychiatric reactions in patients as they wake up from anesthesia. The best anesthetic for ECT continues to be debated.

Because the anesthesia is so brief, typically only 10–15 minutes total, most patients are not intubated. Respiration is maintained with a breathing mask administered by an anesthetist or anesthesiologist.

Developing Countries and ECT for Schizophrenia

ECT use is not limited to industrialized nations and remains remarkably popular in many developing countries. Interestingly, ECT is often used in these countries for treating schizophrenia, sometimes in the first episode (Pompili et al. 2013). Large epidemiological studies suggest that over a lifetime, patients with schizophrenia do better in these countries. Could these more favorable outcomes be due to the more aggressive use of ECT, especially early in the disease course? More research is needed regarding this tantalizing association.

One final thought before we leave this topic. We have organized this chapter around the central ECT dogma that a seizure is essential to the therapeutic effect of the procedure: *a seizure is necessary but not sufficient.* However, a recent small study suggests we should not be so sure. Regenold et al. (2015) reported that 11 patients with treatment-resistant depression (who refused ECT) were given nonconvulsive electrotherapy over several weeks. They were put to sleep and given just slightly less electricity than is typically needed to induce seizures. They showed responses and remissions similar to those seen with ECT, without the typical cognitive declines. Darn! Just when it seemed safe to be overconfident…

What Does ECT Do to the Brain?

Patients conceptualize ECT as resetting or rebooting the brain (Dukakis and Tye 2006). It is as though the procedure erases the problems and lets the brain restart afresh. The experts have different explanations, but the actual curative effect of ECT remains unknown. The patients' explanation may be equally plausible.

Anticonvulsant

With regard to treating depression, one would intuitively assume that there is some aspect of the ECT-induced seizure that "awakens" the brain and restores it to its premorbid well condition. In actuality, it is just the opposite, at least in the short term. Figure 4–6 shows a composite positron emission tomography (PET) scan of 10 patients before and after a course of ECT for depression (Nobler et al. 2001). The most remarkable finding is the decreased metabolism in the prefrontal and parietal regions. In general, the reductions in prefrontal activity correlate with treatment outcome. That is, rather than restoring function and returning the brain to its premorbid state, ECT appears at least acutely to be pushing the brain into a different homeostasis, with many areas of the brain exhibiting decreased function, paradoxically while the patient is free of depression.

Paradoxically, ECT, which produces a seizure, is actually an anticonvulsant in the longer term (Sackeim 1999). By inducing a seizure, ECT actually decreases electrical activity of the brain. If

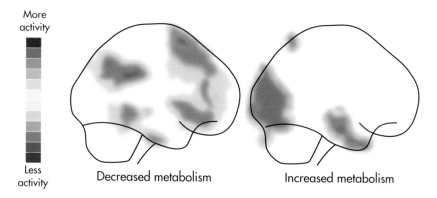

More
activity

Less
activity

Decreased metabolism   Increased metabolism

FIGURE 4-6.   Brain activity following a course of ECT.
Prefrontal and parietal regions show decreased cerebral glucose metabolism after a course of ECT. Relative increases in glucose metabolism were primarily limited to the occipital lobes.
Source.   Adapted from Nobler et al. 2001.

depression is the result of aberrant electrical activity, as some believe, then the antidepressant effect of ECT may be due to its capacity to quiet the brain. By inhibiting electrical activity, or producing a cascade of pharmacological events that the brain naturally uses to stop seizures from spreading, ECT may help the brain to function more efficiently. Others have reformulated this idea to state that depression may be due to hyperconnected, overdriven circuits. ECT may act to stop these pathological hyperconnections and restore normal, more flexible patterns of connection.

Nerve Growth Factors

Animal and human research over the past decade suggests that depression may result from a decrease in nerve growth factors such as brain-derived neurotrophic factor (BDNF) (Higgins and George 2019). The theory proposes that the loss of nerve growth factors such as BDNF results in a decrease in activity in the neural networks involved in mood. Disparate treatments such as the antidepressants, lithium, and exercise all increase BDNF. Furthermore, the stimulation therapies TMS and vagal nerve stimulation (VNS), as well as ECT, also increase BDNF.

So, one possible explanation for the effectiveness of ECT could be that it restores growth factor proteins to normal levels (Bocchio-Chiavetto et al. 2006). The growth factor proteins in turn stimulate neural growth, which could restore normal connections, which, in turn, reinstates normal mood.

Neuroendocrine

Subtle neuroendocrine abnormalities are common among the seriously mentally ill (Wolkowitz and Rothschild 2003). The hypothalamic-pituitary-adrenal (HPA) axis and the thyroid gland are frequently discussed as having links to mood disorders. Max Fink (2001) and others have postulated that ECT works by changing the hormonal balance of the brain. In theory, the ECT-induced seizure causes the release of hormones that are deficient from endocrine glands. The release of the hormones stimulates further production of some as-yet-to-be-identified molecule, which in turn improves the patient's condition.

While the theory has a certain appeal, there is little evidence to support it. No hormone has been identified that would fit this model.

Safety and Adverse Events

Mortality

ECT is relatively safe. However, it is a medical procedure involving repeated sessions of general anesthesia, and there is known morbidity and even, in rare cases, mortality. The mortality rate is estimated to be similar to that for minor surgery or childbirth. The American Psychiatric Association Task Force on Electroconvulsive Therapy (Weiner 2001) estimated a current rate for mortality from ECT as approximately 1 per 10,000 patients or 1 per 80,000 treatments.

Cognitive Impairment

The adverse effects of ECT on cognition are the most troubling aspect of the procedure. The seizure induces an obtunded state from which the patient slowly emerges over minutes to several hours. Some patients, particularly the elderly, fail to clear quickly and can remain in a lingering delirium. Although this is not common, such patients must delay additional treatment until the delirium clears.

For all patients, memories of the events immediately around the procedure are never recovered. In fact, the long-term memories are never created because of the disruptive effects of the seizure. Memories of events prior to the ECT are initially impaired (retrograde amnesia) but return within a matter of weeks. However, concerns about long-term memories remain a point of controversy between the ECT advocates and the antipsychiatry movement.

ECT advocates, typically clinicians who practice the procedure and study the research, conclude that retrograde amnesia is a short-term problem. They believe that ECT does not affect the neural structure of long-term memories. Antipsychiatry enthusiasts, on the other hand, present cases of individuals who experience the troubling inability to recall events from their past even years after the procedure (Breggin 1994).

Unfortunately, hard science on the accuracy of recall of long-term memories after ECT has been limited. It is difficult to measure memory for distant events—which tend to fade with time under the best of circumstances. The development of autobiographical memory interviews that can be individualized to each patient and administered before and after the procedure has provided one measure of long-term memory retention.

Sackeim et al. (2007) measured cognitive effects of ECT in 347 patients treated in seven New York City hospitals. As would be expected, most of these patients displayed significant cognitive impairments immediately after the ECT course was completed. Almost all of the problems resolved within 6 months. However, some patients continued to have deficits in autobiographical memory at the 6-month follow-up. Further analysis indicated that the extent of the remote memory impairment was related to the type of ECT used. The results are shown in Figure 4–7.

This study demonstrates that remote memories, even autobiographical ones, remain impaired up to 6 months after acute ECT

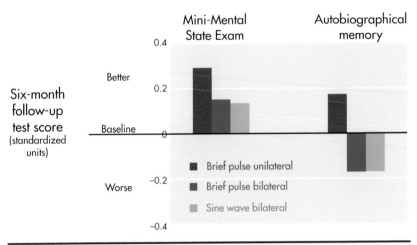

FIGURE 4-7.   Long-term memories after ECT.

For these patients with major depression who were treated with ECT, the Mini-Mental State Examination scores improved from baseline at 6 months. Autobiographical memory scores were worse at 6 months for those patients who received bilateral ECT.

Source.   Adapted from Sackeim et al. 2007.

treatment. The authors noted in their discussion that patients receiving bilateral ECT displayed almost three times the amount of forgetting as that found in the healthy comparison group.

Cardiovascular

There is a high rate of cardiac arrhythmias in the immediate post-ictal period. Most of these events are benign and resolve quickly. Patients with preexisting cardiac disease are at greatest risk for developing irregular rhythms.

Prolonged Seizures

Rare patients will have a prolonged seizure or even status epilepticus. Failure to terminate a persistent seizure not only prolongs the mental confusion after the procedure but also increases the risk of complications from inadequate oxygenation and secondary ischemia.

Headache

The most common physical symptoms after ECT are headaches. As many as 45% of patients complain of a headache. In some, the pain is severe enough to induce nausea and vomiting.

Treatment-Emergent Mania

As with any antidepressant treatment, a small minority of patients will become activated by ECT. It is important to distinguish mania from delirium. If it is mania, some practitioners will continue the treatment because ECT can treat the mania as well. Others will stop the ECT and manage the mania pharmacologically.

Out-of-Date Equipment

Perhaps the greatest safety concern regarding ECT is that some practitioners in the community continue to use outdated equipment and nonstandard treatment protocols (Fink 2007). This results in excessive electrical stimulation that offers no greater benefits but increases the preventable side effects. This may especially be the case in some developing countries, where the procedure can be similar to what Cerletti administered in 1938.

Critical Review of Randomized Controlled Trials of ECT in Neuropsychiatric Applications

Because ECT has been around the longest, it has the largest literature regarding use. It is beyond the scope of this book to review all these studies. Fortunately, the American Psychiatric Association convened a task force, which conducted a thorough review of the literature on the efficacy of ECT and published a report in 2001 (Weiner 2001). Their conclusions on the indications for the use of ECT are summarized here.

Major Depression

Although ECT was initially introduced as a treatment for schizophrenia, the focus of interest quickly moved to patients with mood disorders. Numerous randomized controlled trials have been conducted with ECT in depressed patients. The most remarkable were the trials comparing ECT with sham ECT—a study design that is no longer considered ethical. In the 1940s and 1950s, when ECT was the primary treatment for depression, response rates of 80%–90% were typically reported.

The development of the tricyclic antidepressants (TCAs) and the monoamine oxidase inhibitors (MAOIs) provided alternative treatments for depression and a comparator for ECT. Numerous trials have been conducted comparing ECT with medications and placebo. In a meta-analysis of studies comparing ECT with antidepressants, ECT had a 20% greater response rate compared with TCAs and a 45% greater response rate compared with MAOIs (Janicak et al. 1985). It is worth mentioning that some of the pharmacological treatments in these studies would not be considered adequate medication trials by modern standards.

The task force reviewed other aspects of ECT and concluded that it is effective for

- Bipolar depression.
- Catatonia.
- Psychotic depression.

On the other hand, ECT may be less effective for patients with

- A long duration of current symptoms.
- Depression secondary to medical conditions.
- Those patients with personality disorders.

The current use of ECT in depression is typically reserved for patients who have failed several adequate trials of medication. In these "treatment-resistant" patients, ECT remains the most effective option, but the results are not as robust as those found with treatment-naïve patients. Response rates in patients with treatment-resistant conditions range from 50% to 60%.

To summarize the findings:

- ECT is an efficacious treatment for unipolar and bipolar depression.
- No trial has ever found an alternative treatment superior to ECT.
- ECT is particularly useful in patients with an emergent need for symptom resolution, for example, catatonic and suicidal patients.
- Continuation of some antidepressant treatment after the course of ECT is indicated.

Mania

Prior to the proliferation of antimanic medications, ECT was known to be a fast treatment for mania. Mukherjee et al. (1994) reviewed the literature on ECT in mania and concluded that ECT results in remission or marked clinical improvement in 80% of the cases. However, with the availability of effective antimanic medications, ECT is usually reserved for patients with treatment-resistant mania or those in emergent need of stabilization.

Schizophrenia

Before it became evident that patients with mood disorders were better suited for ECT, many patients with schizophrenia—particularly in public institutions—were given the treatment. The development of antipsychotic medications rapidly altered this practice. However, ECT remains an option for patients who fail to respond to medications.

Current psychiatric practice entails starting patients with schizophrenia on antipsychotic medications. In general, the literature shows that the combination of ECT and antipsychotic medication is superior in outcome to either alone (Weiner 2001). Unfortunately, the definitive randomized trial comparing ECT with and without antipsychotic medications for patients with schizophrenia who fail to respond to medications has yet to be conducted. The question remains: who will benefit from the addition of ECT?

Clearly, some schizophrenia patients improve with the addition of ECT. The literature suggests that patients with a more acute onset of symptoms and of shorter duration are more responsive to ECT. Some clinicians believe that every patient with treatment-resistant schizophrenia deserves at least one full course of ECT, because there will be some who respond to the treatment. They argue that few other options exist for those with chronic, unremitting schizophrenia. A recent study of patients with clozapine-resistant schizophrenia found a 50% response rate with ECT (Petrides et al. 2015).

Parkinson's Disease

ECT can improve general motor function for patients with Parkinson's disease independent of psychiatric symptoms (Weiner 2001). Patients struggling with the "on-off" phenomenon may find particular benefit. Fregni et al. (2005) conducted a recent review of noninvasive brain stimulation for Parkinson's disease and could only find five studies, comprising 49 patients, that met their inclusion criteria. They concluded that ECT appears to have a significant positive effect on motor function in Parkinson's disease patients, but the results should be interpreted with caution because there are only limited studies.

Epilepsy

Paradoxically, ECT can stop a seizure. Since the 1940s, ECT has been known to have anticonvulsant properties (Weiner 2001). During a course of ECT treatment, seizure threshold increases (Sackeim et al. 1983). ECT provides an option for patients with intractable seizures who fail to respond to medications.

Continuation Treatment

Despite the remarkable acute efficacy with ECT, the long-term benefits are difficult to sustain. The relapse rate is particularly high

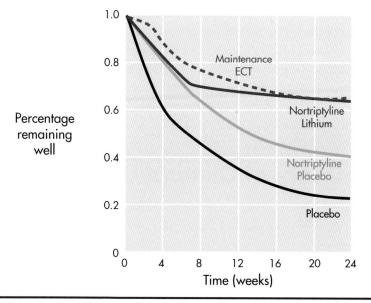

FIGURE 4–8. Six-month relapse rates of patients treated with ECT for depression.

Relapse prevention data after successful ECT for depression highlight the difficulty of keeping people well. Despite limiting enrollment to patients whose depression remitted with ECT and using the best possible therapies for maintenance, the study authors found that almost half the patients relapsed within 6 months. In real-world settings where many patients only experience a partial response, the relapse rates are likely to be even higher.

Source. Data for *solid lines* from Sackeim et al. 2001. Data for *dashed line* from Kellner et al. 2006.

after the sessions are discontinued. The circumstances for major depression are the best studied and provide a good example of the dilemma. The solid lines in Figure 4–8 show the results of a follow-up study of continuation therapy following successful ECT treatment (Sackeim et al. 2001). The authors concluded that without medication virtually all the patients relapsed within 6 months. Monotherapy was marginally effective, but the combination of an antidepressant and lithium provided the best prevention.

Kellner et al. (2006) conducted a similar continuation study but compared maintenance ECT with nortriptyline plus lithium. Maintenance ECT entailed weekly treatments for 4 weeks, biweekly treatments for 8 weeks, and monthly treatments for 2 months. This totaled 10 additional ECT sessions during the 6-month follow-up period. The results are shown with the dashed line in Figure 4–8. The authors concluded that maintenance ECT and the combination of nortriptyline plus lithium were equally effective and equally disappointing. As they noted, "Even more effective strategies for relapse prevention in mood disorders are urgently needed" (Kellner et al. 2006, p. 1337).

Summary of Clinical Use

ECT is the father of the brain stimulation techniques. There has been a slow but important evolution of how ECT is performed, with improvement in response rates and reductions in side effects. Modern ECT with general anesthesia and unilateral ultrabrief pulses is quite different from the ECT Cerletti and others pioneered. However, ECT still carries risks and has cognitive side effects. It is our most effective acute treatment for depression, particularly with psychosis, but the benefits are hard to sustain. It is also useful for acute mania, Parkinson's disease, and status epilepticus.

References

Bocchio-Chiavetto L, Zanardini R, Bortolomasi M, et al: Electroconvulsive therapy (ECT) increases serum brain derived neurotrophic factor (BDNF) in drug resistant depressed patients. Eur Neuropsychopharmacol 16(8):620–624, 2006 16757154

Breggin PR: Toxic Psychiatry: Why Therapy, Empathy and Love Must Replace the Drugs, Electroshock, and Biochemical Therapies of the "New Psychiatry." New York, St. Martin's Press, 1994

Cerletti U: Old and new information about electroshock. Am J Psychiatry 107(2):87–94, 1950 15432756

Dukakis K, Tye L: Shock: The Healing Power of Electroconvulsive Therapy, New York, Avery, 2006

Fink M: Convulsive therapy: a review of the first 55 years. J Affect Disord 63(1–3):1–15, 2001 11246075

Fink M: Improving electroconvulsive therapy practice. Psychiatr Times 24:10–11, 2007

Fitzgerald PB, Hoy KE, Elliot D, et al: A pilot study of the comparative efficacy of 100 Hz magnetic seizure therapy and electroconvulsive therapy in persistent depression. Depress Anxiety 35(5):393–401, 2018 29329499

Fregni F, Simon DK, Wu A, et al: Non-invasive brain stimulation for Parkinson's disease: a systematic review and meta-analysis of the literature. J Neurol Neurosurg Psychiatry 76(12):1614–1623, 2005 16291882

Higgins ES, George MS: The Neuroscience of Clinical Psychiatry: The Pathophysiology of Behavior and Mental Illness, 3rd Edition. Philadelphia, PA, Wolters Kluwer, 2019

Janicak PG, Davis JM, Gibbons RD, et al: Efficacy of ECT: a meta-analysis. Am J Psychiatry 142(3):297–302, 1985 3882006

Kellner CH, Knapp RG, Petrides G, et al: Continuation electroconvulsive therapy vs pharmacotherapy for relapse prevention in major depression: a multisite study from the Consortium for Research in Electroconvulsive Therapy (CORE). Arch Gen Psychiatry 63(12):1337–1344, 2006 17146008

Mukherjee S, Sackeim HA, Schnur DB: Electroconvulsive therapy of acute manic episodes: a review of 50 years' experience. Am J Psychiatry 151(2):169–176, 1994 8296883

Nahas Z, Short B, Burns C, et al: A feasibility study of a new method for electrically producing seizures in man: focal electrically administered seizure therapy [FEAST]. Brain Stimul 6(3):403–408, 2013 23518262

Nobler MS, Oquendo MA, Kegeles LS, et al: Decreased regional brain metabolism after ect. Am J Psychiatry 158(2):305–308, 2001 11156816

Petrides G, Malur C, Braga RJ, et al: Electroconvulsive therapy augmentation in clozapine-resistant schizophrenia: a prospective, randomized study. Am J Psychiatry 172(1):52–58, 2015 25157964

Pompili M, Lester D, Dominici G, et al: Indications for electroconvulsive treatment in schizophrenia: a systematic review. Schizophr Res 146(1–3):1–9, 2013 23499244

Prudic J: Electroconvulsive therapy, in Kaplan and Sadock's Comprehensive Textbook of Psychiatry, 8th Edition. Edited by Sadock BJ, Sadock VA. Philadelphia, PA, Lippincott Williams and Wilkins, 2005

Regenold WT, Noorani RJ, Piez D, et al: Nonconvulsive electrotherapy for treatment resistant unipolar and bipolar major depressive disorder: a proof-of-concept trial. Brain Stimul 8(5):855–861, 2015 26187603

Sackeim HA: Magnetic stimulation therapy and ECT. Convuls Ther 10(4):255–258, 1994

Sackeim HA: The anticonvulsant hypothesis of the mechanisms of action of ECT: current status. J ECT 15(1):5–26, 1999 10189616

Sackeim HA, Decina P, Prohovnik I, et al: Anticonvulsant and antidepressant properties of electroconvulsive therapy: a proposed mechanism of action. Biol Psychiatry 18(11):1301–1310, 1983 6317065

Sackeim HA, Prudic J, Devanand DP, et al: Effects of stimulus intensity and electrode placement on the efficacy and cognitive effects of electroconvulsive therapy. N Engl J Med 328(12):839–846, 1993 8441428

Sackeim HA, Prudic J, Devanand DP, et al: A prospective, randomized, double-blind comparison of bilateral and right unilateral electroconvulsive therapy at different stimulus intensities. Arch Gen Psychiatry 57(5):425–434, 2000 10807482

Sackeim HA, Haskett RF, Mulsant BH, et al: Continuation pharmacotherapy in the prevention of relapse following electroconvulsive therapy: a randomized controlled trial. JAMA 285(10):1299–1307, 2001 11255384

Sackeim HA, Prudic J, Fuller R, et al: The cognitive effects of electroconvulsive therapy in community settings. Neuropsychopharmacology 32(1):244–254, 2007 16936712

Sackeim HA, Prudic J, Nobler MS, et al: Effects of pulse width and electrode placement on the efficacy and cognitive effects of electroconvulsive therapy. Brain Stimul 1(2):71–83, 2008 19756236

Sahlem GL, Short EB, Kerns S, et al: Expanded safety and efficacy data for a new method of performing electroconvulsive therapy: focal electrically administered seizure therapy. J ECT 32(3):197–203, 2016 27379790

Shorter E: A History of Psychiatry, New York, Wiley, 1997

Shorter E: The history of ECT: unsolved mysteries. Psychiatr Times 21(2):93, 2004

Spellman T, Peterchev AV, Lisanby SH: Focal electrically administered seizure therapy: a novel form of ECT illustrates the roles of current directionality, polarity, and electrode configuration in seizure induction. Neuropsychopharmacology 34(8):2002–2010, 2009 19225453

Weiner RD: The Practice of Electroconvulsive Therapy: Recommendations for Treatment, Training, and Privileging—A Task Force Report. Washington, DC, American Psychiatric Publishing, 2001

Wolkowitz OM, Rothschild AJ: Psychoneuroendocrinology: The Scientific Basis of Clinical Practice, Washington, DC, American Psychiatric Publishing, 2003

CHAPTER 5

Vagus Nerve Stimulation

"What happens in Vagus, stays in Vagus. Well, actually, it's just the opposite. The Vagus can't keep a secret."

Introduction and History

The focus of vagus nerve stimulation (VNS) is, of course, the vagus nerve. The vagus nerve, as shown in Figure 5–1, is the tenth cranial nerve and emerges from the brain at the medulla. It is the longest cranial nerve extending into the chest and abdominal cavity. *Vagus* comes from the Latin word for wandering, and this nerve is remarkably complex, both in where it comes from and in the variety of information it passes to and from the brain to the periphery.

Traditionally, the vagus has been conceptualized as modulating the parasympathetic tone of the internal organs. For example, vagal signals from the brain (efferent) are highly active during that wonderful, peaceful time after a good meal. However, most of the signals traveling through the vagus nerve actually go from the organs back into the brain (afferent). Foley and DuBois (1937) established in 1937 that 80% of the signals traveling through the cervical vagus nerve are afferent, while only 20% are efferent.

In 1938, Bailey and Bremer made an important discovery. They stimulated the vagus nerve of cats and reported that this synchronized the electrical activity in the orbital cortex. In 1949, MacLean and Pribram did similar studies with anesthetized monkeys (MacLean 1990). Using electroencephalography, they found that VNS generated slow waves over the lateral frontal cortex. If you think about it, the vagus nerve is to the body what the optic nerve is to the external world. The optic nerve carries information about the external world, whereas the vagus nerve represents the "eyes" into our internal world—our body and basic life processes.

The afferent fibers in the vagus travel to the solitary nucleus and then to the locus coeruleus. Remember that the locus is where all of the norepinephrine cells in the brain originate, and they project diffusely up to the cortex. Other secondary vagus fibers eventually connect to the orbitofrontal cortex and the insula, in somatotopically defined regions. They terminate in areas of the limbic brain, which regulates emotion. It is no surprise then that when we grieve, we have a "broken heart." We actually sense the sensation in our heart because the vagus cardiac fibers terminate in brain regions where the limbic system and gut sensations overlap.

Jake Zabara, in the mid-1980s, was the first to demonstrate convincingly the therapeutic benefits of VNS (Groves and Brown 2005). The story of how Zabara came to discover the therapeutic potential of VNS is another example of serendipity, science, and psychiatric treatment. As he once told the story to one of the authors (M.S.G.), Zabara was studying the vagus nerve when his

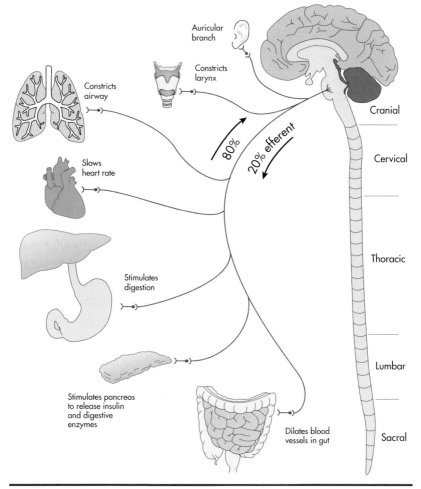

FIGURE 5–1.   The vagus nerve.

The vagus nerve provides parasympathetic innervation from the brain to numerous internal organs (efferent activity). However, most of the electrical activity through the vagus nerve proceeds from the thorax back into the brain (afferent activity). Also, note how the branch to the larynx diverges close to the brain stem—typically, above the placement of the VNS electrode.

wife was pregnant. As a dutiful husband, he attended the Lamaze classes to help his wife master the proper breathing techniques that would assist her through the pain of childbirth. He wondered if the therapeutic benefits of deep and regulated breathing were mediated from the diaphragm through the vagus nerve into the brain.

Zabara began experimenting with dogs. He exposed and stimulated the vagus nerve. One dog developed a seizure, and Zabara was able to stop the seizure by stimulating the vagus nerve. Eureka! Later, Zabara induced seizures in dogs with strychnine and showed that repetitive electrical stimulation of the vagus nerve interrupted the motor seizures. Of particular interest to Zabara was the lasting effect of VNS. That is, the anticonvulsant benefits could outlast the period of stimulation by a factor of four. Constant stimulation was not required for enduring effects.

The first self-contained cervical devices were implanted in humans in 1988 in patients with intractable, medically unresponsive epilepsy. Results were positive and side effects minimal for these difficult-to-treat patients. VNS became available for use in Europe in 1994 and was given a U.S. Food and Drug Administration (FDA) indication for epilepsy in the United States in 1997.

In 1997, Cyberonics Inc., the company with the VNS patent, approached several psychiatric experts and asked if VNS might be useful in mood disorders. Several lines of evidence suggested that VNS might be helpful in patients with depression. While no objective studies had yet been done, there were numerous anecdotal reports of patients with VNS saying they had never felt better in their lives. Furthermore, and perhaps most impressive, functional imaging studies demonstrated that VNS increased activity in several regions of the brain thought to be involved with depression (Figure 5–2) (Henry et al. 1998).

Pilot studies were conducted using VNS with patients who had treatment-resistant depression. Later, Cyberonics sponsored one randomized controlled trial (reviewed later in this chapter). In Europe, VNS was approved for depression in 2001. The FDA approved cervically implanted VNS in 2005 for patients with depression who have failed four adequate trials of medication.

Since the first edition of this book, additional methods have been developed for stimulating the vagus nerve, which requires us to expand our description of VNS. It turns out the vagus nerve does more than communicate with visceral organs below the neck. It also communicates with facial structures such as the larynx,

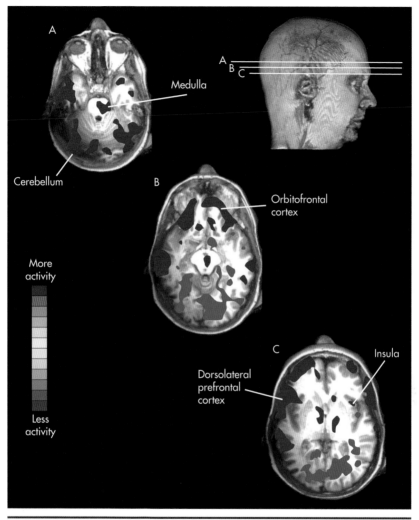

FIGURE 5-2. Effect of VNS on the brain.

Ten patients with VNS treatment for epilepsy underwent positron emission tomography (PET) measurement before and during vagus stimulation. VNS, compared with rest, caused relative activation of areas associated with depression (e.g., dorsolateral prefrontal cortex, insula, orbitofrontal cortex, cingulate gyrus).

Source. Adapted from Henry et al. 1998.

pharynx, and ear. The auricular branch is of particular interest because it can be stimulated by applying electricity directly to the external ear. Consequently, we make a distinction between cervical VNS and transcutaneous auricular VNS (taVNS).

How Is It Done?

There are a variety of ways to stimulate the vagus nerve, but in humans, VNS typically refers to stimulation of the left cervical vagus nerve using a commercially available device that in many ways is similar to a cardiac pacemaker. That is, a battery-operated generator is implanted subcutaneously in the left chest wall, attached to an electrode tunneled under the skin, and wrapped around a nerve. With cervical VNS, the surgeons typically wrap the electrode around the left vagus nerve in the neck (Figure 5–3).

Cervical VNS implantation is usually an outpatient procedure in the United States typically performed by neurosurgeons. The battery in the device generates an intermittent electrical stimulation that is delivered to the vagus nerve. Clinicians following the patient can control the frequency and intensity of the stimulation. Adjustments to the stimulation parameters are transmitted from a computer to the VNS device by a handheld infrared wand placed over the device.

The wire wrapped around the nerve is directional, with clear instructions as to which end should be proximal to the brain. Some speculate that this unidirectional feature helps minimize efferent side effects. However, it is likely that at least some patients have had the leads reversed, without noticeable harm.

Wrapping a Wire Around a Nerve

The cervical vagus nerve is actually a large nerve bundle made up of different-sized nerves going to and from the brain. Some nerves are myelinated and send information quickly; others are naked axons that pass the signals along at a slower pace (Figure 5–4). Some nerves sit close to the outside and are easily accessible to stimulation, whereas others are hidden in the center and are more difficult to reach.

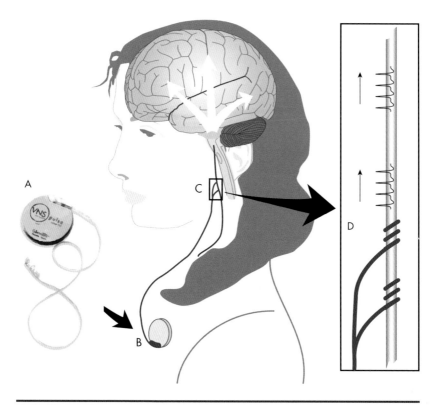

FIGURE 5–3. The commercially available VNS apparatus.
The VNS generator **(A)** contains a small battery that generates electrical impulses. A surgeon implants the device under the skin over the chest **(B)** and attaches the electrodes to the left vagus nerve **(C)**. Regular signals from the VNS device travel up the vagus nerve **(D)** and ultimately alter activity in the cerebral cortex.

The key point is that the vagus nerve is a complex structure. The modern form of cervical VNS can be compared to wrapping a rope around a tree and trying to influence the flow of phloem and xylem in order to change behavior in a particular branch. The relatively crude nature of the intervention does not allow for as precise a stimulation as we would like. Microsurgical techniques might theoretically allow for more focal VNS. Or, as we discuss later, you can find vagus-specific fibers right as they exit a specific organ, such as the stomach, and stimulate only those fibers.

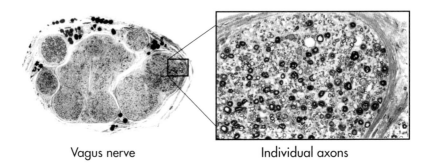

Vagus nerve   Individual axons

FIGURE 5-4.   Cross-section of the vagus nerve.

The vagus nerve contains approximately 100,000 afferent and efferent axons. A closer view shows that most axons are unmyelinated (the dark circles are myelin).

Closed Loop Feedback

There are numerous locations to stimulate the "wandering" vagus nerve. The left side was chosen because of concerns that the right vagus controls the pacemaker regions of the heart. However, some patients with left vagus trauma have had safe VNS of the right side. For epilepsy, the AspireSR and SenTiva VNS therapy systems are the two most recently developed VNS devices. These novel devices have implemented a closed-loop approach and contain a cardiac-based seizure detection algorithm. When a seizure starts, the heart rate skyrockets, and this then automatically triggers the VNS device to send out an extra train of stimulation.

Over the past decade, many researchers have started to get ever more specific in terms of which branches of the vagus to stimulate, how to stimulate noninvasively, or how to pair vagus stimulation with behaviors to reshape the brain and promote learning and plasticity. We tackle these now.

Noninvasive Cervical VNS

One company has developed a method of stimulating the vagus nerve in the neck with a small handheld electrical device that looks roughly like an electric razor. This passes current through the neck tissues, some of which then goes through the vagus. This company, electroCore, calls its device gammaCore. It was FDA approved in

2017 for treating the acute phase of episodic cluster headache. The gammaCore device has not been studied for use with depression.

Auricular Branch

A cutaneous branch of the vagus innervates parts of the ear (auricular branch of the vagus nerve [ABVN]). Could you stimulate the vagus through skin stimulation of the ear (the taVNS)? Does auricular or ear acupuncture or cutaneous stimulation stimulate vagus fibers? Maybe the ancient Chinese acupuncturists knew long ago what we are now rediscovering (Usichenko et al. 2017). Some clinicians argue that the ABVN is a small-diameter nerve and that stimulation cannot carry enough "bandwidth" to enable therapeutic effects. However, recent neurophysiological and imaging studies show that taVNS can activate central vagus fibers in a manner similar to more traditional cervical VNS (Badran et al. 2018a, 2018b). The taVNS devices typically stimulate with an electrode clipped to either the tragus or the cymba conchae of the external ear. Currently, there are no FDA-approved indications for taVNS, although it is an active area of research.

Gastric Vagus

We desperately need better treatments for obesity. Early studies with VNS hinted that it might help with weight management. Some thoughtful clinicians speculated that stimulation of the vagus fibers as they immediately exit the stomach might give a more focused stimulation. The thought being that when the vagus fibers immediately exit from an end organ such as the stomach, you can be reasonably assured that you are just stimulating gastric vagus fibers. Vagus stimulation is a new FDA-approved treatment for obesity.

Other Possibilities

Additionally, there has been much excitement about pairing VNS with behaviors. Apparently, when the vagus is stimulated, it immediately activates norepinephrine fibers, which "wake up" the brain and say, "Pay attention to this!" By pairing either cervical or transcutaneous auricular VNS with tones (tinnitus), physical rehabilitation (motor stroke), speech therapy (aphasia), or sucking a bottle (premature infants learning to feed), one can enhance learning and reinforce a new behavior.

Finally, recent preclinical research reveals that VNS induces effects on brain plasticity, the autonomic nervous system, and the inflammatory response. These findings suggest new indications for VNS, such as stroke rehabilitation, management of chronic heart failure, management of rheumatoid arthritis, and reversal of brain damage after cardiac arrest. The utility of VNS stimulation keeps expanding.

Dosing

How much stimulation is needed with VNS to get an effect? Actually, this has never been completely explored and likely depends on the VNS method and the behavior or disease you are trying to influence. The original dosing parameters (e.g., intensity, frequency, duration) for cervical VNS were established by Jake Zabara when he experimented with dogs. He induced experimental seizures in dogs and found dosing parameters that were effective at stopping most of the seizures. Primarily for safety reasons, those same parameters are largely what are still in use today. A thorough analysis of dosing and response for various disorders has yet to be conducted, with the exception of recent dosing parametric studies for taVNS (Badran et al. 2018a, 2018b).

The initial cervical epilepsy studies compared two dosing parameters—high stimulation and low stimulation (see Table 5–1). The low-stimulation group was believed to be receiving subtherapeutic stimulation and therefore functioned as a control group.

The present version of the generator (B in Figure 5–3) can be programmed for the following domains: intensity, pulse width (130, 250, 500 microseconds), frequency (1, 20, 30 Hz), on time, and off time. Unfortunately, the delivery has to follow these strict rules and cannot be "intermittent." That is, one cannot have the device fire for only a few hours per day or have variations in the delivered dose. This is unfortunate, because with intermittent dosing you could have the device fire only during sleep, or at specific times of the day, timed perhaps with circadian changes. We know that the brain quickly adapts to consistent stimuli but has trouble

TABLE 5–1. Stimulation parameters for high-dose and low-dose groups in the original epilepsy trials of VNS

	High stimulation	Low stimulation
Frequency	30 Hz	1 Hz
Pulse width	500 microseconds	130 microseconds
Length of stimulation	30 seconds "on"	30 seconds "on"
Length of time between stimulations	5 minutes "off"	90–180 minutes "off"
Total vagus electrical stimulation per day	**129.6 seconds/day**	**0.047 seconds/day**

Note. The high-stimulation group received more stimulation, more frequently (approximately 2,500 times as much!).

adapting to variety. It will be interesting to watch as this area progresses whether intermittent stimulation has profoundly different biological properties.

A series of studies with VNS inside the functional magnetic resonance imaging (fMRI) scanner has shown that varying these parameters changes which brain regions are affected. Different pulse widths, frequencies, and intensities all result in varying maps of VNS effects in the brain. It is clear that by altering the electrical pulse in the neck, you can change the major brain regions affected by VNS. Unfortunately, this fine-tuning has not yet made it into clinical practice.

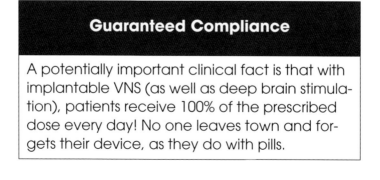

Guaranteed Compliance

A potentially important clinical fact is that with implantable VNS (as well as deep brain stimulation), patients receive 100% of the prescribed dose every day! No one leaves town and forgets their device, as they do with pills.

Emergency Shutoff

For cervical VNS, each patient is given a magnet that, when held over the device, will immediately shut off stimulation. Consequently, patients have the ability to turn off the device temporarily to eliminate troublesome side effects. For example, some patients wish to stop the voice tremor during public speaking. When the magnet is removed, normal programmed stimulation quickly resumes. Patients who wish to shut off stimulation for extended periods of time must find ways to secure the magnet directly over the device until they are ready to resume treatment.

What Does VNS Do to the Brain?

Cervical VNS has antiseizure and neuropsychiatric effects. How cervical VNS alters the brain and produces these effects is a matter of speculation. Some of the theories are reviewed in the following discussion. End organ–specific VNS, such as gastric VNS for obesity, simply sends vagus signals to the brain artificially (e.g., falsely making you think that your stomach is full and you should eat less!).

"Bottom-Up" Stimulation

Electroconvulsive therapy (ECT) and transcranial magnetic stimulation (TMS) are stimulation therapies that originate at the top of the brain (outer cortical mantle) and work their way down. VNS, on the other hand, is a "bottom-up" therapy, with information flow beginning in the cranial nerve and then the brainstem. The afferent signals coming up the vagus nerve relay information to the nucleus tractus solitarius (NTS) in the medulla (Figure 5–5). The NTS relays the signal through several pathways, perhaps the most important of which goes through the locus coeruleus. These signals are in turn relayed to higher areas of the brain, as shown in the functional imaging studies in Figure 5–2.

Changing Rhythms

Some authors have suggested that VNS controls seizures by changing the electrical rhythms of the brain. We mentioned that early researchers noted slowing on the electroencephalogram (EEG) (not in humans) with vagus stimulation. This may be accom-

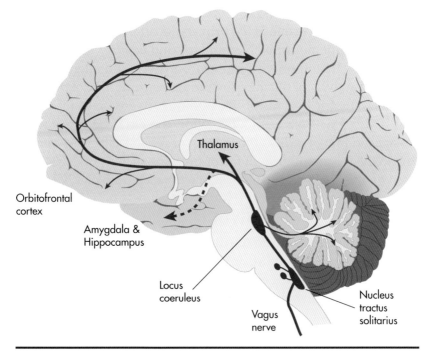

FIGURE 5–5. Vagus nerve afferent connections.

The afferent fibers of the vagus nerve terminate in the nucleus tractus solitarius, which has connections with the locus coeruleus (and several other structures, such as the raphe nuclei). Projectors from the locus coeruleus to other areas of the brain are believed to mediate the effects of VNS.

plished through stimulation of the ascending reticular activating system, which projects to numerous forebrain structures (Amar et al. 1998). Interestingly, VNS does not readily change the EEG in humans, although it does in other animals. This has frustrated efforts to accurately understand how VNS works and adjust the dose for patients. One of the more common theories about how VNS works is that it may affect the thalamus and alter the rhythmic firing of the thalamus and cortex (thalamocortical firings). This theory has not been proven.

Norepinephrine

The locus coeruleus clearly plays a vital role in the effectiveness of VNS. Lesions of the locus coeruleus in rats eliminate the ability of

VNS to suppress seizures. The locus coeruleus is also of particular interest because it is one of the primary locations for cell bodies of norepinephrine neurons. Norepinephrine activity is altered by medications that improve depression, anxiety, and attention. The enhanced activity of the norepinephrine neurons may explain the neuropsychiatric benefits of VNS. Numerous studies have found that if you pair VNS with a behavior, the brain becomes more plastic and more readily able to learn or rehabilitate. This may be due to the release of growth factor proteins such as BDNF stimulated by the norepinephrine release with each train of VNS.

Gamma-Aminobutyric Acid

Gamma-aminobutyric acid (GABA) is the primary inhibitory neurotransmitter in the brain. Anticonvulsants such as valproate, phenobarbital, and the benzodiazepines exert their antiseizure effects in part by enhancing GABA. It is also well known that many anticonvulsants have psychiatric benefits in addition to controlling seizures.

VNS appears to enhance GABA activity (Groves and Brown 2005). VNS has been shown to increase the free GABA in the cerebrospinal fluid. Additionally, responders to VNS have been shown to have increased GABA receptor density. It is possible that VNS reduces seizure activity by increasing GABA and the inhibition of the brain.

Alternative Medicine

Some speculate that the calming feature of such activities as yoga and chanting are mediated through vagus stimulation. A recent study of experienced yoga practitioners showed that 1 hour of yoga increased the brain GABA levels by 27% (Streeter et al. 2007). Only further research will tell if these changes are induced through the vagus nerve.

Continued Improvement With Time

One of the most unique features of cervical VNS for epilepsy and depression (see Figure 5–6 later in the chapter) is the enhanced efficacy with continued use over time. That is, more patients respond at 12 months than at 3 months. Importantly, once one responds to VNS, the effects often last for many years (Aaronson et al. 2017). This suggests that vagus stimulation gradually changes something in the brain. Just as with exercise and weight loss, the results are not immediate.

As we discussed in Chapter 4, VNS, as well as ECT, increases BDNF. VNS might help the brain through its gradual effects on growth factors such as BDNF, which in turn "repair" the damaged brain.

Safety and Adverse Events

The adverse events associated with VNS are best separated into those associated with the complications of the surgery and those resulting from the side effects of stimulation.

Surgical Complications

The risks associated with cervical VNS surgery are minimal (O'Reardon et al. 2006). As with most surgical procedures, those surgeons who are more skilled will have fewer complications and better results. Wound infections are infrequent (less than 3%) and are managed with antibiotics. Pain at the surgical site almost always resolves within 2 weeks. Rarely, left vocal cord paresis persists after surgery (<1 in 1,000), but this usually resolves slowly over the ensuing weeks.

Temporary asystole during the initial testing of the device is a rare but serious surgical complication. In approximately 1 out of 1,000 cases, asystole has been reported in the operating room during initial lead testing. It may be a result of aberrant electrical stimulation resulting from poor hemostatic control. That is, blood in the surgical field causes arcing of the current, and the cardiac branch gets depolarized. Fortunately, no deaths have been reported because normal cardiac rhythm has always been restored. Postoperatively, these patients have been able to safely use VNS. More importantly, no cardiac events have been reported when the device is turned on for the first time after surgery.

Physical Side Effects From Stimulation

After the initial testing in the operating room, the patient is typically allowed to heal for 2 weeks before the stimulator is again turned on. The most common side effects are associated with stimulation and thus only experienced when the device is on. Hoarseness, dyspnea, and cough are the most common side effects. They appear to correlate with stimulation intensity and can be minimized with reductions in the stimulation parameters. Some people do not like the feeling of the generator under the skin on their chest. One fellow said it felt like a tuna can on his chest. Newer devices are smaller.

Most cervical VNS side effects decrease with time. Hoarseness or voice alteration is the most persistent problem. Between 30% and 60% of patients continue to experience this side effect during times of stimulation, although for reasons that are unclear this also diminishes over months to years.

Parasympathetic Response?

One would speculate that cervical VNS might increase the impulses going down the vagus nerve to the internal organs and induce a parasympathetic response. However, this has not been an issue. Vital signs have remained stable with cervical VNS. Cardiac slowing has not been a problem. This may be due to the placement of the leads above the branches from the vagus nerve going to the heart. In contrast, transient heart rate reductions are typically seen with auricular VNS. VNS also has been investigated as a treatment for congestive heart failure.

> ## Parasympathetic Response? *(continued)*
>
> Stimulation of the vagus can definitely change the heart, but it depends on which branch of the vagus that is stimulated as well as the parameters that are used (e.g., intensity, pulse width, frequency, duty cycle).

Psychiatric Side Effects

As with any effective treatment for depression, unintended manic activation is a worrisome side effect. Hypomania and frank mania have been reported (1%–3%) with cervical VNS. Usually these symptoms developed in patients with a prior diagnosis of bipolar disorder. Reducing the intensity of the stimulation or adding a mood-stabilizing agent is the best way to manage the symptoms.

Emergence of suicidal ideation is a concern with antidepressants but has not been a problem with cervical VNS. Likewise, cognitive impairment has not been an issue, and actually, many patients report improved cognitive function (Sackeim et al. 2001). The lack of cognitive impairment is one advantage in using VNS in children with epilepsy. Most of the anticonvulsant medications induce cognitive slowing or a feeling of sluggishness, both of which impede learning.

Critical Review of Randomized Controlled Trials of VNS in Neuropsychiatric Applications

FDA approval for stimulation therapies is different than what is done for medications. With stimulation procedures, the FDA approves (or technically "clears") the device for a specific disease. So only one patented device has received FDA approval for cervical VNS, even though many devices could potentially deliver similar impulses. Additionally, the FDA does not require as many trials or as many patients studied to receive approval for a device as it requires for medications.

Epilepsy

There have been two large, acute, double-blind, controlled studies of cervical VNS in patients with treatment-resistant epilepsy (Ben-Menachem et al. 1994; Handforth et al. 1998). As described earlier, low stimulation served as the control in comparison to high stimulation. In this difficult-to-treat population, seizure frequency decreased 28%–31% in the high-stimulation group compared with baseline while only dropping 11%–15% in the low-stimulation group.

Unfortunately, few patients were able to stop their anticonvulsant medications. However, many were able to reduce the number of medications they took per day—which likely improves cognitive processing and learning, especially important in children.

Long-term follow-up studies show the typical pattern for VNS: that is, continued improvement up to 1 year and then stabilization of effect. There appears to be no tolerance to VNS. The patient with the longest exposure to VNS has had the system operating for more than 20 years. Although initially slow to be accepted, cervical VNS has assumed a small but significant role in epilepsy practice.

A new advance in cervical VNS for epilepsy is the closed loop system in which the device can be automatically triggered by a rapid increase in heart rate, suggesting a seizure has started.

Depression

The situation with depression is more complicated. Initial pilot studies with 59 patients with treatment-resistant depression demonstrated good results—30% response rate at 10 weeks. Even more encouraging were the extended results. Patients continued to improve after the acute phase of the trial. Patients were actually doing better at 1 year than they were at 3 months (Figure 5–6). This is a rare pattern in the treatment of depression.

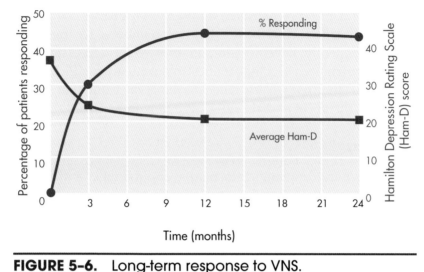

FIGURE 5–6. Long-term response to VNS.

Follow-up analysis of the original 59 VNS patients showed continued improvements up to 1 year and sustained benefits up to 2 years.

Results from a pivotal multicentered, randomized, double-blinded trial of VNS were not as encouraging. In this trial, active VNS failed to statistically separate from sham treatment. The response rates for the acute treatment of treatment-resistant depression were 15% for active treatment and 10% for sham treatment (Rush et al. 2005).

A parallel but nonrandomized group was also studied and compared with those patients who received VNS in this pivotal trial. Thus, one group received the addition of VNS and the other received "treatment as usual." They were followed for 12 months, during which time both groups received similar treatment (medications and ECT) except for the VNS difference. At the end point the response rates were significantly different: 27% for the VNS group and 13% for the treatment-as-usual group (George et al. 2005).

The FDA considered all these studies when evaluating VNS for depression. They were most impressed with the long-term enduring benefits for this difficult-to-treat population. In 2005, they approved VNS for patients with chronic or recurrent depression, either unipolar or bipolar, with a history of failing to respond to at least four antidepressant trials. However, this is not Class I evidence (a positive double-blind, placebo-controlled study). Most insurance companies demand Class I evidence before they will reimburse for treatment and, consequently, have not jumped on VNS for depression. Recently there has been increased interest in potentially conducting another Class I trial, particularly given the remarkable durability of the device (Aaronson et al. 2013, 2017). We remain hopeful.

Obesity

The vagus nerve transmits information about hunger and satiety from the gut to the brain. Could stimulating the vagus nerve fool the brain into thinking the body is full? This is an exciting prospect that could potentially treat the epidemic of obesity. Early studies with dogs demonstrated significant changes in eating behavior as well as weight loss with vagus stimulation subdiaphragmatically (Roslin and Kurian 2001).

For humans, a device has been developed that stimulates vagus fibers right as they exit from the stomach. This is called a vagal block, or VBLOC. Unlike VNS in the neck, this device only interacts with vagus fibers going to and from the stomach, so right at the organ. Presumably, because of this, the signal traveling up the vagus nerve is more specific to the gut and food intake. The device is inserted below the diaphragm using a laparoscope, so the surgery is less invasive than gastric bypass surgery. It is usually an outpatient procedure. In a large, pivotal trial, 239 obese patients were randomly assigned to receive active (162) or sham (77) VBLOC. After 1 year of stimulation for 12 hours per day, the active patients had an average 28% weight loss—50% more weight loss than the sham group (Ikramuddin et al. 2014). This is an exciting new advance in brain stimulation therapies and shows the power of this new approach with difficult-to-treat conditions.

Cluster Headache

The gammaCore device (the handheld device applied to the neck by the patient) reduces cluster headaches—another difficult-to-treat condition. Two trials of the noninvasive cervical VNS device found that 47% of gammaCore patients were headache pain–free after a treatment as opposed to 6% with sham—a very large effect (Nesbitt et al. 2015).

Anxiety

William James argued that all anxiety resides not in the brain, but rather in the periphery. The James-Lange theory of emotion posited that we are anxious when we see a charging bull not because of our cognitions about a bull, but rather because our heart races and our lungs need air. Although this debate about the origins of anxiety and emotion is still not settled, most believe that anxiety results from both central sources and peripheral sensations, all of which are carried through the vagus nerve. Theoretically, VNS could be a powerful anxiolytic. However, there have not been any controlled trials and only one open clinical trial. Hopefully more research will be done in this application now that there are noninvasive VNS methods.

Pain

The vagus nerve carries pain fibers from the gut and then innervates regions involved in pain perception, such as the insula. It is thus natural to ask whether VNS can affect pain perception. Jeff Borckardt took VNS-implanted patients and hooked them up to devices that could measure their pain thresholds (Borckardt et al. 2005, 2006). Different VNS parameters caused an acute improvement in pain thresholds. There are also case series in which VNS has helped with chronic pain. This is an interesting area for future work, especially in light of the opioid epidemic.

Other

There are ongoing clinical trials pairing cervical VNS with tinnitus (Borland et al. 2018; Engineer et al. 2015, 2017; Tyler et al. 2017), aphasia, and motor stroke recovery (Dawson et al. 2016; Ganzer et al. 2018; Hays et al. 2016). The main company here is Microtransponder.

Dr. Doe Jenkins, working with us, is using taVNS in newborns to see if she can improve and accelerate the very first motor task we must learn: how to suck milk. VNS also has important anti-inflammatory effects, and studies in animals show VNS can stop septic shock as well as preserve brain tissue acutely after stroke (Huston et al. 2007; Ottani et al. 2009). It will be exciting to see over the next decade how many different ways clinicians tap into the healing powers of the vagus nerve.

Summary of Clinical Use

Invasive cervical VNS is a safe and effective treatment for epilepsy. It appears to work in all forms of epilepsy. It is especially useful in pediatric epilepsy, because the device does not have cognitive side effects.

There are two positive open studies of invasive cervical VNS in depression, although the prospective double-blind study did not yield statistically significant results. Uncontrolled long-term studies suggest that the device may be remarkably durable in patients with treatment-resistant depression. Noninvasive cervical VNS can have impressive benefits for those with cluster headaches. Finally, minimally invasive gastric VNS, or VBLOC, is FDA approved for treating morbid obesity. Reasoning from the known anatomy of the vagus, VNS may ultimately have clinical utility for the treatment of many other behaviors such as pain, anxiety, tinnitus, stroke recovery, or even acute treatment of sepsis or brain damage.

References

Aaronson ST, Carpenter LL, Conway CR, et al: Vagus nerve stimulation therapy randomized to different amounts of electrical charge for treatment-resistant depression: acute and chronic effects. Brain Stimul 6(4):631–640, 2013 23122916

Aaronson ST, Sears P, Ruvuna F, et al: A 5-year observational study of patients with treatment-resistant depression treated with vagus nerve stimulation or treatment as usual: comparison of response, remission, and suicidality. Am J Psychiatry 174(7):640–648, 2017 28359201

Amar AP, Heck CN, Levy ML, et al: An institutional experience with cervical vagus nerve trunk stimulation for medically refractory epilepsy: rationale, technique, and outcome. Neurosurgery 43(6):1265–1276, discussion 1276–1280, 1998 9848840

Badran BW, Dowdle LT, Mithoefer OJ, et al: Neurophysiologic effects of transcutaneous auricular vagus nerve stimulation (taVNS) via electrical stimulation of the tragus: a concurrent taVNS/fMRI study and review. Brain Stimul 11(3):492–500, 2018a 29361441

Badran BW, Mithoefer OJ, Summer CE, et al: Short trains of transcutaneous auricular vagus nerve stimulation (taVNS) have parameter-specific effects on heart rate. Brain Stimul 11(4):699–708, 2018b 29716843

Bailey P, Bremer F: A sensory cortical representation of the vagus nerve: with a note on the effects of low blood pressure on the cortical electrogram. J Neurophysiol 1(5):405–412, 1938

Ben-Menachem E, Mañon-Espaillat R, Ristanovic R, et al: Vagus nerve stimulation for treatment of partial seizures: 1. A controlled study of effect on seizures. Epilepsia 35(3):616–626, 1994 8026408

Borckardt JJ, Kozel FA, Anderson B, et al: Vagus nerve stimulation affects pain perception in depressed adults. Pain Res Manag 10(1):9–14, 2005 15782242

Borckardt JJ, Anderson B, Andrew Kozel F, et al: Acute and long-term VNS effects on pain perception in a case of treatment-resistant depression. Neurocase 12(4):216–220, 2006 17000590

Borland MS, Engineer CT, Vrana WA, et al: The interval between VNS-tone pairings determines the extent of cortical map plasticity. Neuroscience 369:76–86, 2018 29129793

Dawson J, Pierce D, Dixit A, et al: Safety, feasibility, and efficacy of vagus nerve stimulation paired with upper-limb rehabilitation after ischemic stroke. Stroke 47(1):143–150, 2016 26645257

Engineer CT, Engineer ND, Riley JR, et al: Pairing speech sounds with vagus nerve stimulation drives stimulus-specific cortical plasticity. Brain Stimul 8(3):637–644, 2015 25732785

Engineer CT, Shetake JA, Engineer ND, et al: Temporal plasticity in auditory cortex improves neural discrimination of speech sounds. Brain Stimul 10(3):543–552, 2017 28131520

Foley JO, DuBois F: Quantitative studies of the vagus nerve in the cat. I. The ratio of sensory and motor studies. J Comp Neurol 67(1):49–67, 1937

Ganzer PD, Darrow MJ, Meyers EC, et al: Closed-loop neuromodulation restores network connectivity and motor control after spinal cord injury. eLife March 2018 29533186 Epub

George MS, Rush AJ, Marangell LB, et al: A one-year comparison of vagus nerve stimulation with treatment as usual for treatment-resistant depression. Biol Psychiatry 58(5):364–373, 2005 16139582

Groves DA, Brown VJ: Vagal nerve stimulation: a review of its applications and potential mechanisms that mediate its clinical effects. Neurosci Biobehav Rev 29(3):493–500, 2005 15820552

Handforth A, DeGiorgio CM, Schachter SC, et al: Vagus nerve stimulation therapy for partial-onset seizures: a randomized active-control trial. Neurology 51(1):48–55, 1998 9674777

Hays SA, Ruiz A, Bethea T, et al: Vagus nerve stimulation during re-habilitative training enhances recovery of forelimb function after ischemic stroke in aged rats. Neurobiol Aging 43:111–118, 2016 27255820

Henry TR, Bakay RA, Votaw JR, et al: Brain blood flow alterations induced by therapeutic vagus nerve stimulation in partial epilepsy: I. Acute effects at high and low levels of stimulation. Epilepsia 39(9):983–990, 1998 9738678

Huston JM, Gallowitsch-Puerta M, Ochani M, et al: Transcutaneous vagus nerve stimulation reduces serum high mobility group box 1 levels and improves survival in murine sepsis. Crit Care Med 35(12):2762–2768, 2007 17901837

Ikramuddin S, Blackstone RP, Brancatisano A, et al: Effect of reversible intermittent intra-abdominal vagal nerve blockade on morbid obesity: the ReCharge randomized clinical trial. JAMA 312(9):915–922, 2014 25182100

MacLean PD: The Triune Brain in Evolution. New York, Plenum, 1990

Nesbitt AD, Marin JC, Tompkins E, et al: Initial use of a novel noninvasive vagus nerve stimulator for cluster headache treatment. Neurology 84(12):1249–1253, 2015 25713002

O'Reardon JP, Cristancho P, Peshek AD: Vagus nerve stimulation (VNS) and treatment of depression: to the brainstem and beyond. Psychiatry (Edgmont Pa) 3(5):54–63, 2006 21103178

Ottani A, Giuliani D, Mioni C, et al: Vagus nerve mediates the protective effects of melanocortins against cerebral and systemic damage after ischemic stroke. J Cereb Blood Flow Metab 29(3):512–523, 2009 19018269

Roslin M, Kurian M: The use of electrical stimulation of the vagus nerve to treat morbid obesity. Epilepsy Behav 2(3):11–16, 2001

Rush AJ, Marangell LB, Sackeim HA, et al: Vagus nerve stimulation for treatment-resistant depression: a randomized, controlled acute phase trial. Biol Psychiatry 58(5):347–354, 2005 16139580

Sackeim HA, Keilp JG, Rush AJ, et al: The effects of vagus nerve stimulation on cognitive performance in patients with treatment-resistant depression. Neuropsychiatry Neuropsychol Behav Neurol 14(1):53–62, 2001 11234909

Streeter CC, Jensen JE, Perlmutter RM, et al: Yoga Asana sessions increase brain GABA levels: a pilot study. J Altern Complement Med 13(4):419–426, 2007 17532734

Tyler R, Cacace A, Stocking C, et al: Vagus nerve stimulation paired with tones for the treatment of tinnitus: a prospective randomized double-blind controlled pilot study in humans. Sci Rep 7(1):11960, 2017 28931943

Usichenko T, Hacker H, Lotze M: Transcutaneous auricular vagal nerve stimulation (taVNS) might be a mechanism behind the analgesic effects of auricular acupuncture. Brain Stimul 10(6):1042–1044, 2017 28803834

CHAPTER 6

Transcranial Magnetic Stimulation

Introduction and History

Transcranial magnetic stimulation (TMS) involves inducing an electrical current within the brain using pulsating magnetic fields that are generated outside the brain near the scalp. It is important to understand that TMS is not simply applying a static or constant magnetic field to the brain. Our man in Figure 6–1 is holding a magnet against his head. Although static powerful magnets can subtly affect his brain, it is certainly not conventional TMS. To understand TMS, we must review some basic electromagnetic principles.

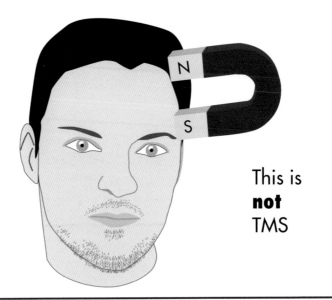

FIGURE 6–1. Man holding a magnet to his head.

The constant magnetic force does not produce any electrical pulse. Our current knowledge suggests that the effects of a constant magnetic field on the brain are minimal. The important aspect of TMS is the electrical current induced in the brain by the pulsing magnetic field.

By 1820, scientists discovered that passing an electric current through a wire induces a magnetic field. This has become a common grade school science experiment. Students wrap a wire around a nail and attach each end to a battery, turning that nail into an electromagnet (see Figure 2–2). It was Michael Faraday in 1832 who discovered that the inverse was also true.

Faraday showed that passing a magnet through a coil generates an electrical current. Figure 6–2 shows an example of this process. We need to remember that the current is only generated while the magnet is passing through the coil. It is the *changing magnetic field* that generates the electricity. A static magnet resting inside the coil will not generate a current.

An electromagnet offers an alternative way to create a changing magnetic field and thus induce an electrical pulse. An intermittent electrical signal will generate an intermittent magnetic pulse. It is the pulsating magnetic field that induces an electrical current (Figure 6–3). So, in essence, the electrical current from a wall socket can

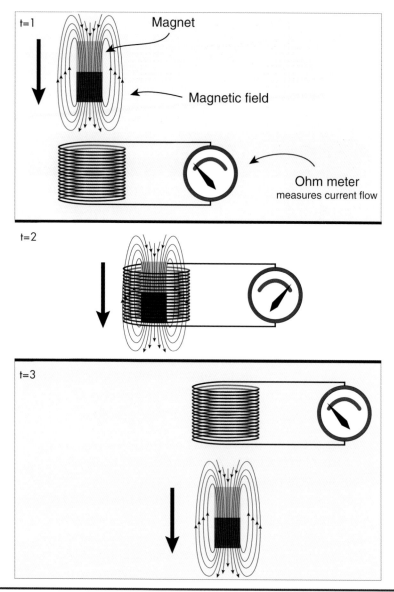

FIGURE 6-2. Faraday's law.

Passing a magnet through a coil generates an electrical current. This is the basis of hydroelectric power plants (water turns a magnet in a coil, producing electricity). It is also the basis of TMS. t=time.

generate a magnetic field, which is pulsated and can then induce an electrical signal. And, as we have discussed in previous chapters, focally applied electricity can have powerful effects on the brain. For most TMS applications, it likely is the electricity induced from the pulsating magnet, and not the magnetic field itself, that has the profound and sometimes therapeutic effects on the brain.

Animal Magnetism

There is a long history of dubious claims about the healing power of magnets (Shermer 2002). One of the earliest and most famous examples is the claim made by the German physician Franz Anton Mesmer, who in 1775 introduced the term "animal magnetism." Mesmer believed that humans possess an invisible magnetic field whose properties were altered in the physically ill. For a time, he aroused considerable interest in his magnetic cures—passing magnets over the bodies of patients to alter their magnetic fields. Benjamin Franklin, commissioned by the King of France, helped debunk Mesmer's claims.

More recently, there has been a resurgence of interest in magnets. A quick search of the internet reveals numerous companies offering magnetic shoe insoles, belts, mattress pads, and so on that are purported to relieve pain and suffering. A review of the available scientific literature on studies with static magnets finds little evidence supporting benefits of this therapy (Ratterman et al. 2002). In contrast, however, there are reputable studies showing that holding a powerful (2T) magnet on the skull for 20 minutes can change the underlying excitability of the brain, but without proven therapeutic benefits.

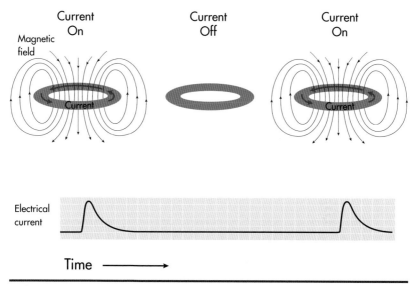

FIGURE 6-3. Electromagnetic induction.

An electrical current induces a magnetic field in the coil. Turning the magnetic field on and off induces an electrical change in the area around the coil.

The first known examples of anything close to modern TMS occurred in the years 1910 and 1911 (George and Belmaker 2007). At that time, several researchers used large magnets the size of suitcases (or even trunks) to induce phosphenes: the sensation of seeing light without actual light passing into the eye. It is unclear from that work whether the magnets stimulated the retina or the occipital cortex. These early experiments were fascinating but of little practical value. Interest in the field waned for many decades.

In 1959, Kolin and his colleagues demonstrated that a fluctuating magnetic field could stimulate a peripheral frog muscle in preparation. However, it was not until 1985 that the modern era of TMS started. That year, Anthony Barker in Sheffield, England, described the use of a noninvasive magnetic device resembling modern TMS instruments (Barker et al. 1985). The device was slow to recharge and quick to overheat, but it was a start.

Does TMS Really Change Brain Activity?

One of the most troubling questions for many skeptical scientists and clinicians regarding TMS is: can an electromagnet really affect the brain? Four quick points establish that TMS has profound and easily observable effects on the brain.

1. TMS of the motor cortex will induce corresponding muscle contractions in the appropriate arm or leg.

2. Seizures are a real but rare side effect of TMS.

3. Placing an active coil over the occipital cortex will induce visual sensations.

4. Repetitive TMS over Broca's area will induce temporary aphasia.

The first attempts to use repetitive TMS (rTMS) as treatment were with depressed patients. In the early 1990s, George—working in Robert Post's lab at the National Institute of Mental Health—wrote the first paper and described in detail the outcome for one patient with treatment-resistant depression who received daily prefrontal rTMS. Figure 6–4 shows the patient's Hamilton Depression Rating Scale score over the course of three TMS treatment phases.

This case report is particularly interesting because the authors, with all due respect, did not necessarily know what they were doing. Like Cerletti with electroconvulsive therapy (ECT), they were making educated guesses about the best way to administer a new treatment. Research suggested that left prefrontal cortex (PFC) dysfunction plays a significant role in depression, so they placed the coil over the left PFC.

How many sessions of TMS are needed to treat depression? Figure 6–4 shows that the researchers underestimated the amount

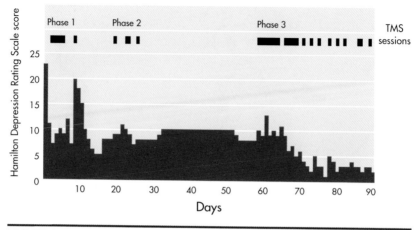

FIGURE 6–4. Early TMS experience.

A case study showing one women's response to repeated daily prefrontal TMS in the early days of its use.

Source. Adapted from George et al. 1995.

needed in the first two treatment phases for this patient. It was not until after the extended third treatment course that the patient achieved remission. Once again, we see that the parameters of a new treatment are often only uncovered through trial and error, especially if there are no easy animal surrogates to determine dose.

How Is It Done?

TMS requires a big machine and looks more like something one would find in a dental office. As with any device that advertises therapeutic benefit, the U.S. Food and Drug Administration (FDA) marshals control. The devices are regulated for general safety, and the companies can only advertise for approved disorders. In the United States, seven devices have received FDA clearance for treating depression, with the first approval going to Neuronetics in 2008 (O'Reardon et al. 2007). The Neuronetics apparatus is used to illustrate the process of TMS in Figure 6–5. As discussed before, the essential feature is using electricity to gen-

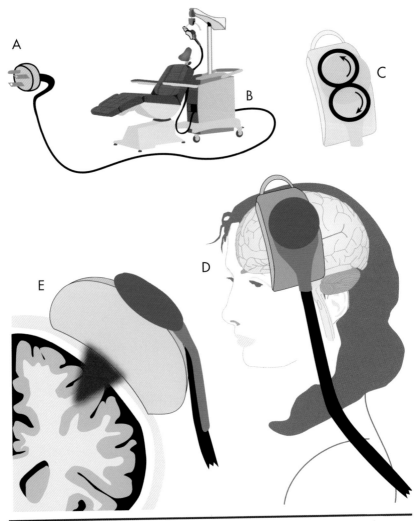

FIGURE 6–5.   A TMS machine and how it is commonly used to treat depression.

Alternating current from the wall **(A)** is used to charge a bank of large capacitors **(B)**. A pulsating electrical current generated in coils inside the device **(C)** produces a pulsating magnetic charge. The patient reclines in the chair, and the TMS coil is placed over his or her left prefrontal cortex **(D)** or other regions. The electrical charge is rapidly discharged through the magnetic coil and induces a magnetic field that travels through the skin and skull. This fluctuating magnetic field in turn induces an electrical current in brain areas just below the skull, depicted in **(E)**.

TABLE 6–1. Examples of common magnetic force in tesla

Example	Force (in tesla)
Earth's magnetic field	0.00005
Refrigerator magnet	0.1
12-volt battery nail electromagnet	0.5
Magnetic resonance imaging (MRI)	3
Transcranial magnetic stimulation (TMS)	1.5–3
World's strongest magnet (Florida State)	45

erate a rapidly changing magnetic field, which in turn produces an electrical impulse in the brain.

The common unit of magnetic field strength is the *tesla*, denoted "T," equal to 1 Newton/1 ampere×1 meter [N/(A×m)] (Force/Current-Distance); one T is about 20,000 times the Earth's magnetic field. Technically, TMS devices produce a fairly powerful magnetic field, but only very briefly. Table 6–1 shows examples of common magnetic forces for comparison.

Early TMS devices only emitted a single, brief pulse. Modern devices can generate a rapid succession of pulses, called *repetitive TMS* (rTMS). The typical treatment for depression is a 20- to 40-minute session, 5 days a week for 4–6 weeks. To keep the patient still and the device correctly placed, the patient is instructed to recline in a chair and the device is held securely against his or her head (see Figure 6–5).

The TMS coil (encased in plastic housing in Figure 6–5C) generates a magnetic field impulse that can only reach the outer layers of the cortex. Some devices are single coils, whereas others are two coils side by side (also called a "figure eight"). The impulse may only go 2–3 centimeters below the device. Deeper focused noninvasive penetration is the holy grail of TMS research.

Deeper Signal

The Brainsway company has built a device that can send a deeper and broader electrical signal. While it can stimulate around the nucleus accumbens, the pleasure center, there is no evidence that the stimulation is actually pleasurable. This is fortunate, as such a device might be popular at college parties, and it already looks like the user is wearing a lampshade. The FDA might then have to step in and regulate this as a "controlled device," analogous to a "controlled substance." And we already have enough government regulation as it is! Unfortunately, it is not clear that deeper penetration results in better clinical effects. Figure 6–6 shows the Brainsway device (A) and the coils inside the device (B).

Motor Threshold

When the TMS device produces a pulse over the motor cortex, a volley of electrochemical activity descends through the brain, into the spinal cord, and out the peripheral nerve, where it can ultimately cause a muscle to twitch. The minimum amount of energy needed to observe the contraction of the thumb (abductor pollicis brevis) is called the *motor threshold*. This is used as a measure of general cortical excitability (see discussion later). A percentage of the motor threshold serves as a safe and effective setting for rapid TMS (e.g., 120% of motor threshold).

Although this convention has helped make TMS safer, it is severely insufficient in that it is referenced only to each machine and thus is not a universal quantifiable measurement of dose. Future work is focusing on more universal, constant measures of the magnetic field delivered.

Frequency

In general, with TMS, a stronger, more intense pulse results in more activation of the central nervous system tissue and a wider area of

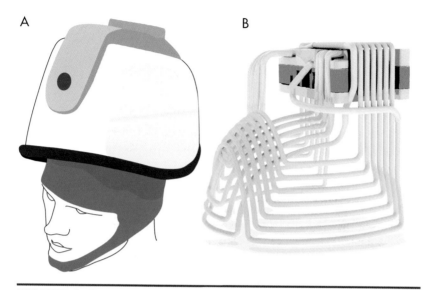

FIGURE 6-6. Brainsway device with deeper and broader electrical signal.
(A) Illustration of device. (B) Coils inside the device.

activation. Frequency is a bit different. Different frequencies can have opposite effects. In general, frequencies of less than 1 per second (<1 Hz) are actually inhibitory (Hoffman and Cavus 2002). This may be because low-frequency TMS more selectively stimulates the inhibitory gamma-aminobutyric acid (GABA) neurons.

Another interesting frequency is a complex pattern called *theta burst*. If we were to put an electrode into the hippocampus and listen, we would hear neurons "chirping" with a theta burst pattern. For many years, neuroscientists have known that stimulating nerve cells with theta burst was the most powerful way to change firing patterns and modulate circuits either through long-term depression or long-term potentiation. The theta "burst" is a triplet at 50 Hz, repeated at 5 Hz (hence the term *theta*). Constant theta burst (cTBS) is, in general, inhibitory, whereas intermittent theta burst (iTBS) is excitatory.

The ability to focally inhibit or excite various regions of the brain sets the stage for the amazing number of clinical trials using TMS. While most uses of TMS seek to activate the brain, some disorders, such as epilepsy, panic disorder, and hallucinations, likely result from neural hyperactivation and would need low-frequency TMS or cTBS. Having an instrument to cool off these neurons could be of potential value for patients with such conditions.

Home TMS

A handheld device developed by Neuralieve is now FDA approved to abort migraine headaches. The device delivers a single large pulse. When the patient experiences the aura phase of an impending headache, he or she holds the device to the back of the head and directs the pulse toward the occipital cortex. The pulse attempts to extinguish the migraine when it is still small, before it gets out of control. The beauty of the device is that patients can have it with them and use it when they sense a headache brewing.

Spinning Magnets

While a static magnet will not induce electrical currents in the brain, you could spin a round magnet right next to the skull. This would produce a changing magnetic field and, as Dr. Faraday would quickly remind us, induce current to flow in the brain. This is precisely what one company, called Neosync, has done. They have a device that spins three different round magnets positioned in the midline of the head. The spin rate is the patient's alpha frequency, which varies from person to person but is usually in the range of 8–12 Hz. This company has completed one positive clinical trial, with another under way. Because the induced currents are not powerful enough to depolarize a neuron, this device cannot cause a seizure and likely could be used at home.

What Does TMS Do to the Brain?

The conventional TMS device interacts with and generally activates the cortex immediately underneath the site of administration. This effect has been shown repeatedly with functional imaging studies. Although the direct stimulation of deep brain regions is out of reach for most machines, secondary activation of deeper structures is a feature of the procedure. Figure 6–7 shows the cortical activation of

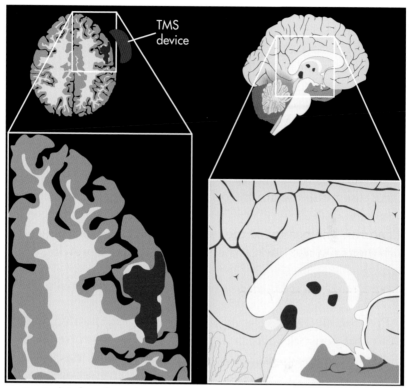

Cortical: Left prefrontal cortex   Subcortical: Thalamus

FIGURE 6-7. Effects of TMS on the brain.

A TMS device placed over the left prefrontal cortex actives the gray matter directly underneath the coil as well as deeper subcortical structures that are beyond the direct reach of the TMS signal.

Source. Adapted from Li et al. 2004.

the left PFC directly below the TMS coil and the indirect subcortical activation of the thalamus (Li et al. 2004).

The effects of TMS pulses on the neuron are inadequately understood. We believe that the electrical impulse generates an action potential in the neurons that it can reach. The action potential runs down the neuron and can excite other neurons. The net result is that numerous downstream brain structures are affected. The problem is that within any section of cortex, there are local inhibitory neurons as well as excitatory neurons that send signals elsewhere. Which neurons are excited or inhibited depends on several factors such as orientation of the fibers, intensity, and frequency, to name just a few. It is unclear exactly how best to deliver TMS to selectively activate different neuronal elements.

When treating depression, TMS most likely activates the PFC, which initiates a cascade of signals to other regions of the brain. These signals increase or decrease activity in cortical and subcortical areas that are connected to the networks of the PFC. Just as a TMS pulse to the motor cortex will trigger a distant twitch in the corresponding muscle, so will a pulse to the PFC induce downstream neural effects. Some of these effects appear to modulate the neural systems that alleviate depression and pain.

At a molecular level, TMS is known to have effects similar to those seen with ECT:

- Increased monoamine turnover
- Increased brain-derived neurotrophic factor
- Normalization of the hypothalamic-pituitary-adrenal axis

Presumably TMS exerts its effects on the brain through the activation of networks, which in turn change gene expression, resulting in changes to the molecular environment of the CNS. For example, recent work has shown that a successful antidepressant course of TMS causes an increase in the size of the anterior cingulate cortex. We assume that TMS induces gene expression of growth factor proteins like BDNF, and this in turn increases dendritic branching and synapse formation, which increases the size of the gray matter in the anterior cingulate.

Safety and Adverse Events

In general, TMS is regarded as safe and without enduring side effects. There have been no reported lasting neurological, cognitive, or cardiovascular sequelae as a result of TMS. However, TMS can alter brain function, so we must remain vigilant about the possible development of long-term problems.

Seizures

Inducing a seizure is the primary safety concern with TMS. There have been at least 200 published TMS-induced seizures, but we do not know how many unpublished seizures occurred. Since we do not know the total number of TMS sessions that have been performed, we cannot produce an accurate estimate of the frequency. However, we believe the incidence of seizures is rare (George and Belmaker 2007; Rossini et al. 2015). There are no reports of TMS causing recurrent seizures, and all of the seizures occurred during TMS administration when the patient was sitting down and near an investigator. Also, all of the seizures were self-limited without needing medications or significant interventions.

Of the reported cases, the majority of the patients were receiving TMS to the motor cortex—the most epileptogenic region of the cortex. Additionally, most (but not all) were receiving trains of stimulation outside of suggested limits. These cases suggest that TMS-induced seizures will remain a rare but significant adverse event even in patients without histories of seizures and even when TMS is used within suggested guidelines.

Hearing Loss

One patient reported temporary hearing loss after TMS. In light of this, an extensive study of auditory threshold was conducted before and after 4 weeks of TMS in more than 300 patients. No changes were found. None of the TMS coils exceed hearing safety guidelines, but as a general precaution patients and treaters are advised to wear earplugs or earbuds during treatments (Perera et al. 2016).

Headache

Mild headaches are the most common complaint after TMS, in up to 20% of some studies. These are generally treated with aspirin and other over-the-counter analgesics.

Cognitive Impairment

Analysis of neurocognitive functioning of TMS patients has not found any enduring negative effects from the procedure. After a session, patients are able to drive home and return to work.

Critical Review of TMS in Neuropsychiatric Applications

TMS has been tested as a treatment in numerous conditions (Perera et al. 2016; Ridding and Rothwell 2007). Presumably TMS has the potential not only to change the immediate electrical activity in the cortex in close proximity to the magnet but also to induce alterations in more distant neural structures that will endure beyond the sessions. This issue is addressed in the conditions discussed in the following subsections.

Depression

Depression has been the most widely studied condition with TMS. Figure 6–4 shows one of the early case studies. Not shown is the dramatic awakening the procedure produced in the patient's positron emission tomography scan at the end of the study. So, not only did the patient feel better, but she had convincing objective evidence to show that her brain was more active. Results such as this stimulated numerous controlled studies. George and other neuropsychiatrists identified the left PFC as a potential treatment target for depression. Converging lines of evidence from functional neuroimaging experiments, stroke studies, and the stimulation location producing optimal response to ECT, as well as animal studies, suggested the left PFC was a good place to focus treatment. In 1995, these researchers demonstrated that over the course of daily TMS sessions, high-frequency (20-Hz) stimulation for 800 total pulses per session, applied over the presumed location of the left PFC (approximately 5 cm anterior to the motor cortex) at an intensity of 80% of the resting motor threshold (rMT) significantly improved depressive symptoms in two of six patients with medication-resistant depression (George et al. 1995). While these results were revelatory, larger clinical evaluations of TMS using sham-controlled designs were still necessary to pin down the ideal stimulation parameters, including the standardization of how to determine the stimulation target in the PFC, the number of pulses to apply within each TMS session, the intensity of stimulation, and how to individually dose the intensity of the treatment.

The most rigorous clinical test of prefrontal TMS for treating depression was the National Institutes of Health–funded, industry-independent OPT-TMS trial (George et al. 2010). This multisite, sham-controlled trial enrolled 190 patients who had medication-resistant depression (as defined by inadequate response to two or more pharmacological therapies) in a 3-week-duration adaptive-treatment design. Participants who had a 30% or greater improvement in depression during the fixed treatment period, whether from active or from sham stimulation, continued their treatment condition for up to 3 weeks longer, while those with a lower than 30% improvement exited to receive active TMS treatment without breaking the blind concerning their initial treatment. The researchers acquired an rMT (the amount of stimulation to cause a muscle twitch 50% of the time) for each participant on a weekly basis, and the treatment was administered at 120% of the rMT to ensure that stimulation was delivered suprathreshold. In each session, stimulation was applied at 10 Hz (10 pulses per second) for 4 seconds, with 26 seconds between each stimulation train (grouping of TMS pulses), for a total of 3,000 pulses per session. The stimulation target was 5 or 6 cm anterior to the scalp location of the rMT. The primary and secondary outcomes were the number of patients who achieved remission or had a response to the treatment (defined by a Hamilton Depression Rating Scale score of 3 or less or a 50% or greater reduction in score, respectively).

The study designers were especially concerned about the placebo control. Prior to this study, even the best sham systems did not control for the differential pain of stimulation, the noise induced by the coils, or the "twitch" of scalp muscles underneath the coil. Any competent treater could quickly figure out which patients were getting real or sham treatment. Thus, unblinded treaters were in the same room as the patients for as long as 30 hours. The OPT-TMS study perfected a new form of sham that mimicked the pain and produced the same twitch (Borckardt et al. 2006, 2008, 2009). Both patients and treaters wore noise-canceling earbuds.

At the conclusion of the study the rates of remission and response were significantly higher in the active treatment condition compared with the sham treatment (14.1% vs. 5.1% for remission; 15% vs. 5% for response). Further analyses showed that active stimulation participants were 4.2 times more likely to reach remission and 4.6 times more likely to fulfill response criteria.

The open-label trial following the acute double-blind phase also yielded positive results, with 29.9% of patients reaching remission (Mantovani et al. 2012; McDonald et al. 2011). Notably, this cohort comprised active and sham participants, with the remitters being almost equivalently from each group (30.2% from the active TMS condition and 29.6% from the sham TMS condition), suggesting that prolonged treatment can lead to improved outcome even for those individuals not initially having a robust response to TMS.

The finding that active TMS to the left PFC had greater remission and response rates than sham stimulation firmly contributed to the body of literature that has now led to FDA approval of TMS for depression for first one device (developed by Neuronetics [O'Reardon et al. 2007]) and, more recently, six more (developed by Brainsway [Levkovitz et al. 2015], Magstim, MagVenture, Nexstim, Neurosoft, and Mag & More). There are now likely more than 50 TMS manufacturers around the world.

There is ongoing discussion about the ways to optimize TMS treatment for depression. Drawing on findings of chronic hyperactivation in the right PFC due to depression, some researchers have suggested that an alternative to high-frequency, excitatory TMS over the left PFC would be to stimulate using low-frequency (1-Hz), inhibitory TMS over right prefrontal areas. A growing body of evidence supports this treatment strategy (Klein et al. 1999), although it has not yet been included in the FDA-cleared treatment parameters. Other TMS treatment protocols using high-frequency stimulation have safely altered the parameters without affecting treatment efficacy, using higher-frequency (18-Hz) stimulation with shorter trains (2 seconds) and intertrain intervals (20 seconds) and fewer total pulses per session (1,980 pulses) (Levkovitz et al. 2015). Further investigations into other pulsed pattern stimulation methods, such as theta burst stimulation (TMS delivered in bursts of three 50-Hz pulses at the theta frequency of 5 Hz), and their effect on cortical activation, are in progress (Huang et al. 2005), with promising early results reported (Williams et al. 2018). Blumberger and colleagues (2018) recently completed a large randomized but not controlled or blinded trial comparing theta-burst TMS with conventional 10-Hz TMS. The theta-burst treatment only takes 3 minutes, compared with almost 30 minutes for the standard treatment. The two treatments did not differ. This research has started to change how TMS is delivered clinically, as the theta-burst treatments take less time and clinicians can treat more patients per day.

Obsessive-Compulsive Disorder

One manufacturer has obtained FDA approval for marketing a TMS device for treating obsessive-compulsive disorder (OCD). Brainsway (mentioned earlier in this chapter with regard to deep brain stimulation) designed a special coil that can stimulate the cingulate cortex, one of the regions implicated in OCD. Treatment consists of brain stimulation with psychotherapy.

Patients start by meeting with a psychologist before the treatment course and list a hierarchy of different compulsions or obsessions. Then, across the different days of treatment, the TMS treater has the patient remember and focus on a compulsion right before the treatment begins, and then during the session. This application highlights the trend of formally manipulating the state of the brain during TMS (Adams et al. 2014).

Schizophrenia

Auditory hallucinations are part of the positive symptoms of schizophrenia. These types of hallucinations are believed to result from aberrant activation of the language perception area at the junction of the left temporal and parietal cortices (Higgins and George 2019). Low-frequency TMS could potentially inhibit this area in patients with schizophrenia and provide relief from auditory hallucinations.

A recent meta-analysis looked at the efficacy of low-frequency TMS as a treatment for resistant auditory hallucinations in schizophrenia (Aleman et al. 2007). The authors found 10 sham-controlled studies involving 212 patients. Their review concluded that TMS was effective in reducing auditory hallucinations. Unfortunately,

TMS had no effect on other positive symptoms or the cognitive deficits of schizophrenia. Larger studies are needed to definitely establish the efficacy, tolerability, and utility of TMS for schizophrenia.

There have been four randomized controlled trials of intermittent daily prefrontal TMS to treat negative symptoms in patients with schizophrenia. Only one of these studies was positive.

Tinnitus

Tinnitus is a common, often disabling disorder for which there is no adequate treatment. As many as 8% of adults age 50 years or older have tinnitus, which can often be quite distressing. Recent functional imaging studies have identified increased activity in the auditory cortex in patients with tinnitus.

Low-frequency TMS offers a possible mechanism to "cool off" the overactive auditory cortex that may be producing tinnitus. Several small, controlled trials from one research group in Germany have produced impressive results. Unfortunately, a large, multicenter study failed to find an effect of TMS on tinnitus (Landgrebe et al. 2017).

Pain

Numerous small, controlled studies have evaluated the utility of TMS in patients with pain (George and Belmaker 2007). Studies suggest TMS over either the motor cortex or PFC can provide pain relief in diverse pain conditions. In a clever study of patients recovering from gastric bypass surgery, 20 minutes of real or sham TMS was administered to the PFC of every patient. Subsequently, patients' use of self-administered morphine was followed over the next 48 hours. Those receiving real TMS used 40% less of the medication (Figure 6–8).

Subsequent studies showed that TMS can be beneficial for chronic pain. Repeated sessions of PFC or motor cortex rTMS over several weeks have found effective pain reductions that generally persist for several months (Borckardt et al. 2014; Short et al. 2011; Taylor et al. 2013; Umezaki et al. 2016).

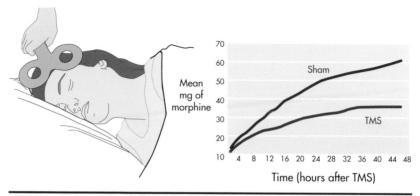

FIGURE 6–8. TMS for pain relief.

Twenty minutes of TMS delivered immediately postoperatively reduced the use of morphine by 40%.

Source. Adapted from Higgins and George 2019.

Headache

The handheld device developed by Neuralieve, mentioned earlier in this chapter, is FDA cleared as a treatment for migraine headaches.

Stroke

Following an ischemic event to the motor cortex, the brain attempts to reorganize the damaged networks. Indeed, the extent of reorganization correlates with the clinical recovery of motor function. TMS may accelerate the reorganization process and therefore enhance recovery.

Different types of TMS may be beneficial in stroke recovery. High-frequency TMS to the affected area may enhance reorganization. Alternatively, low-frequency TMS to the opposite, intact hemisphere is believed to reduce the interference from the non-stroke side. Some believe that too much input from the unaffected side of the brain impedes recovery. Reducing excitability with low-frequency TMS may enhance recovery. The trials so far have been disappointing.

Posttraumatic Stress Disorder

Exposure therapy is the gold standard for treating posttraumatic stress disorder (PTSD). However, some patients do not respond to this treatment or do not want to dredge up what they are trying to forget. There are several small trials using TMS in conjunction with exposure therapy as a way to accelerate the healing process. Small studies stimulating over either the right or the left PFC have shown some positive results. Pivotal industry-sponsored trials are under way.

Addictions

There are some single-site clinical trials showing therapeutic effects of TMS for treating the addictions. Again, most studies combine TMS with some form of cue-induced craving while the patient is in the chair in order to activate the brain regions they are trying to change.

Research Uses

TMS has great potential for basic science research, not just treatment applications. Because of its noninvasiveness and relatively favorable safety profile, TMS is actively used to help us understand the functional mechanisms of the brain. The other brain stimulation techniques, because of their invasiveness and safety concerns, would never be used as a primary research tool. Although a full review is beyond the scope of this book, we can outline these broad areas here.

Physiology. Delivered over the motor system, TMS can provide a range of relevant information about how excitable a section of brain is. So far, we can only study this over motor cortex, where we measure the peripheral effects of stimulation by examining the responses in muscles (local and distributed motor cortex physiology). When you stimulate the motor cortex, you can make the thumb move and can measure the amount of muscle contraction by hooking the thumb to an oscilloscope (called the *motor evoked potential* [MEP]). Using the MEP, you can determine the 1) motor threshold and 2) cortical silent period or 3) cortical excitability using paired-pulse TMS.

The *cortical silent period* is the amount of time it takes a muscle to return to its resting state after it has been made to discharge with TMS. With *paired-pulse TMS,* researchers apply two pulses through the same coil in quick succession. By varying the time between pulses, or the relative strength of the first pulse compared with the second, one can minimize or enhance the second MEP. These three approaches can be used to understand the cortical effects of central nervous system–active medications (for review, see Ziemann 2003) or to understand how different behaviors change cortical excitability. They can also be used to investigate different disease states.

Interruption–speech arrest. An entirely separate area of research involves using TMS to produce interruption of a behavior. This can be seen while using TMS over the motor cortex for the hand. While the TMS coil is discharging, it is difficult, if not impossible, to use the same hand for anything else. The intermittent TMS firing causes the hand to be clumsy and uncoordinated.

A similar phenomenon occurs when you place a TMS coil over Broca's area (involved in speech production). If the subjects are asked to speak, the moment the TMS coil is over the correct area, they experience an immediate (and fortunately temporary) speech aphasia. Although they can say some syllables, they are not able to say the proper words. In their internal voice, they are talking perfectly. This speech arrest is a dramatic demonstration of the power of TMS to influence circuits. It has been suggested that every clinician treating stroke patients should participate in such an experiment so they can appreciate the frustration of being aphasic.

Influencing or biasing. Cognitive neuroscientists are using TMS to tease out the mechanisms of some behaviors. For example, one group has shown that single pulses of TMS at the right time at specific locations can alter how a person responds to a choice between two objects. With a pulse, the subject chooses A; without a pulse, B is chosen. Some have gone so far as to call this "mind control." However, such research helps cognitive neuroscientists understand the regional activity involved in specific behaviors.

Summary of Clinical Use

TMS offers a noninvasive, safe mechanism to influence brain activity. TMS is FDA cleared for treating the acute phase of depression, with most work focusing on treatment-resistant depression. It is now also FDA-cleared for treating OCD. There are also some trials suggesting potential uses for hallucinations in schizophrenia, pain, tinnitus, PTSD, and the addictions. Future work will involve establishing better parameters (intensity, duration, and location) to enhance the effectiveness and utility of TMS.

References

Adams TG Jr, Badran BW, George MS: Integration of cortical brain stimulation and exposure and response prevention for obsessive-compulsive disorder (OCD). Brain Stimul 7(5):764–765, 2014 25048526

Aleman A, Sommer IE, Kahn RS: Efficacy of slow repetitive transcranial magnetic stimulation in the treatment of resistant auditory hallucinations in schizophrenia: a meta-analysis. J Clin Psychiatry 68(3):416–421, 2007 17388712

Barker AT, Jalinous R, Freeston IL: Non-invasive magnetic stimulation of human motor cortex. Lancet 1(8437):1106–1107, 1985 2860322

Blumberger DM, Vila-Rodriguez F, Thorpe KE, et al: Effectiveness of theta burst versus high-frequency repetitive transcranial magnetic stimulation in patients with depression (THREE-D): a randomised non-inferiority trial. Lancet 391(10131):1683–1692, 2018 29726344

Borckardt JJ, Smith AR, Hutcheson K, et al: Reducing pain and unpleasantness during repetitive transcranial magnetic stimulation. J ECT 22(4):259–264, 2006 17143157

Borckardt J, Walker J, Branham RK, et al: Development and evaluation of a portable sham transcranial magnetic stimulation system. Brain Stimul 1(1):52–59, 2008 19424444

Borckardt JJ, Linder KJ, Ricci R, et al: Focal electrically administered therapy: device parameter effects on stimulus perception in humans. J ECT 25(2):91–98, 2009 19092677

Borckardt JJ, Reeves ST, Kotlowski P, et al: Fast left prefrontal rTMS reduces post-gastric bypass surgery pain: findings from a large-scale, double-blind, sham-controlled clinical trial. Brain Stimul 7(1):42–48, 2014 24527503

George MS, Belmaker RH: Transcranial Magnetic Stimulation in Clinical Psychiatry. Washington, DC, American Psychiatric Publishing, 2007

George MS, Wassermann EM, Williams WA, et al: Daily repetitive transcranial magnetic stimulation (rTMS) improves mood in depression. Neuroreport 6(14):1853–1856, 1995 8547583

George MS, Lisanby SH, Avery D, et al: Daily left prefrontal transcranial magnetic stimulation therapy for major depressive disorder: a sham-controlled randomized trial. Arch Gen Psychiatry 67(5):507–516, 2010 20439832

Higgins ES, George MS: The Neuroscience of Clinical Psychiatry: The Pathophysiology of Behavior and Mental Illness. Philadelphia, PA, Wolters Kluwer, 2019

Hoffman RE, Cavus I: Slow transcranial magnetic stimulation, long-term depotentiation, and brain hyperexcitability disorders. Am J Psychiatry 159(7):1093–1102, 2002 12091184

Huang Y-Z, Edwards MJ, Rounis E, et al: Theta burst stimulation of the human motor cortex. Neuron 45(2):201–206, 2005 15664172

Klein E, Kreinin I, Chistyakov A, et al: Therapeutic efficacy of right prefrontal slow repetitive transcranial magnetic stimulation in major depression: a double-blind controlled study. Arch Gen Psychiatry 56(4):315–320, 1999 10197825

Kolin A, Brill NQ, Broberg PJ: Stimulation of irritable tissues by means of an alternating magnetic field. Proc Soc Exp Biol Med 102:251–253, 1959

Landgrebe M, Hajak G, Wolf S, et al: 1-Hz rTMS in the treatment of tinnitus: a sham-controlled, randomized multicenter trial. Brain Stimul 10(6):1112–1120, 2017 28807845

Levkovitz Y, Isserles M, Padberg F, et al: Efficacy and safety of deep transcranial magnetic stimulation for major depression: a prospective multicenter randomized controlled trial. World Psychiatry 14(1):64–73, 2015 25655160

Li X, Nahas Z, Kozel FA, et al: Acute left prefrontal transcranial magnetic stimulation in depressed patients is associated with immediately increased activity in prefrontal cortical as well as subcortical regions. Biol Psychiatry 55(9):882–890, 2004 15110731

Mantovani A, Pavlicova M, Avery D, et al: Long-term efficacy of repeated daily prefrontal transcranial magnetic stimulation (TMS) in treatment-resistant depression. Depress Anxiety 29(10):883–890, 2012 22689290

McDonald WM, Durkalski V, Ball ER, et al: Improving the antidepressant efficacy of transcranial magnetic stimulation: maximizing the number of stimulations and treatment location in treatment-resistant depression. Depress Anxiety 28(11):973–980, 2011 21898711

O'Reardon JP, Solvason HB, Janicak PG, et al: Efficacy and safety of transcranial magnetic stimulation in the acute treatment of major depression: a multisite randomized controlled trial. Biol Psychiatry 62(11):1208–1216, 2007 17573044

Perera T, George MS, Grammer G, et al: The Clinical TMS Society consensus review and treatment recommendations for TMS therapy for major depressive disorder. Brain Stimul 9(3):336–346, 2016 27090022

Ratterman R, Secrest J, Norwood B, et al: Magnet therapy: what's the attraction? J Am Acad Nurse Pract 14(8):347–353, 2002 12242851

Ridding MC, Rothwell JC: Is there a future for therapeutic use of transcranial magnetic stimulation? Nat Rev Neurosci 8(7):559–567, 2007 17565358

Rossini PM, Burke D, Chen R, et al: Non-invasive electrical and magnetic stimulation of the brain, spinal cord, roots and peripheral nerves: Basic principles and procedures for routine clinical and research application. An updated report from an I.F.C.N. Committee. Clin Neurophysiol 126(6):1071–1107, 2015 25797650

Shermer M: Mesmerized by magnetism. An 18th-century investigation into mesmerism shows us how to think about 21st-century therapeutic magnets. Sci Am 287(5):41, 2002 12395724

Short EB, Borckardt JJ, Anderson BS, et al: Ten sessions of adjunctive left prefrontal rTMS significantly reduces fibromyalgia pain: a randomized, controlled pilot study. Pain 152(11):2477–2484, 2011 21764215

Taylor JJ, Borckardt JJ, Canterberry M, et al: Naloxone-reversible modulation of pain circuitry by left prefrontal rTMS. Neuropsychopharmacology 38(7):1189–1197, 2013 23314221

Umezaki Y, Badran BW, DeVries WH, et al: The efficacy of daily prefrontal repetitive transcranial magnetic stimulation (rTMS) for burning mouth syndrome (BMS): a randomized controlled single-blind study. Brain Stimul 9(2):234–242, 2016 26597930

Williams NR, Sudheimer KD, Bentzley BS, et al: High-dose spaced theta-burst TMS as a rapid-acting antidepressant in highly refractory depression. Brain 141(3):e18, 2018 29415152

Ziemann U: Pharmacology of TMS. Suppl Clin Neurophysiol 56:226–231, 2003 14677399

CHAPTER 7

Deep Brain Stimulation and Cortical Stimulation

Introduction and History

Ablative neurosurgery for movement and psychiatric disorders was relatively common in the 1950s and 1960s (Wichmann and Delong 2006). The development of stereotactic techniques provided greater accuracy and more consistent results for some disorders for which there was little other treatment available. Results were generally positive, although the overuse of frontal lobotomies and

other neurosurgical approaches greatly inhibited growth and research in this field.

The goal of neurosurgery for movement disorders was to remove or isolate an overactive region of the brain. For example, removing part of the ventral intermediate nucleus of the thalamus
was found to improve Parkinson's disease. For psychosurgery, the
objective was the disruption of the offending networks. The frontal lobotomy was believed to isolate the inappropriate signals from
the frontal cortex.

The development of levodopa dramatically reduced the need
for neurosurgical treatments for movement disorders. Likewise,
antipsychotic medications offered new hope for psychiatric patients and accelerated deinstitutionalization. The cavalier imple-
mentation of the frontal lobotomy for the seriously mentally ill
turned public acceptance away from neurosurgery for psychiatric
conditions. It was many years before invasive neurosurgical treatments regained partial favor for psychiatric disorders. The number
of ablative neurosurgeries done for psychiatric patients remains
fewer than 1,000 per year worldwide (Spangler et al. 1996).

The recent resurgence of interest in direct manipulation of the
brain as a viable treatment for movement and psychiatric disorders is the result of two developments. First, pharmacological
treatments were found to be imperfect and often complicated by
side effects. Second, the development of small, battery-operated,
programmable stimulation devices connected to thin leads in the
brain allowed treatment without destroying tissue.

The first implantable cardiac pacemaker was installed in 1958
in Sweden (Nicholls 2007). Although originally designed to simply increase the pace of a bradycardic heart, it has evolved into a
device that can sense inappropriate rhythms and respond accord-
ingly. In 1980, the first cardioverter-defibrillator was implanted.
Such devices detect tachycardias and shock the heart back into a
normal rhythm. Many of these are silent, except when they detect
an abnormal electrocardiographic pattern. This concept is called
responsive stimulation.

In the mid-1980s, Benabid et al. (1993) in France were using
brain stimulation to map the best location to remove the ventral
intermediate nucleus of the thalamus for Parkinson's disease and

essential tremors. Like Penfield before them (see Chapter 1), they used brain stimulation to locate the most appropriate section to remove. They noted that acute stimulation of the ventral intermediate nucleus at frequencies above 60 Hz suppressed the tremors. Furthermore, the effects were lost when the stimulation was stopped. In 1987, they began pilot studies of chronic stimulation for patients who had already been thalamotomized on one side (Benabid et al. 1993). With positive results, they began bilateral stimulation, and this approach is now approved by the U.S. Food and Drug Administration (FDA).

The FDA also approved deep brain stimulation (DBS) in 1997 as a treatment for essential tremor. The FDA has now approved DBS for epilepsy, dystonia, and obsessive-compulsive disorder (OCD). The indications for dystonia and OCD are only "compassionate use" approvals, meaning there are no positive randomized controlled trials and implantation has to be done for patients who have failed other treatments. DBS allows reversible neurosurgical interventions with fewer neurological complications than ablative resection. Theoretically, if the stimulation does not work, you can simply withdraw the thin wire and the brain is largely back where it started. Obviously, you cannot undo resective surgery.

How Is It Done?

Deep Brain Stimulation

The DBS devices are made up of three components: the impulse generator, the extension, and the electrode (see Figure 7–1). The impulse generator is a battery-operated device placed subcutaneously, usually below the clavicle (although some generators are small enough to rest in a cavity in the skull). As with the vagus nerve stimulation (VNS) device, a clinician can externally calibrate the generator to optimize the benefits and minimize the side effects. The extension transmits the electrical signal from the impulse generator to the electrodes. The probes are usually placed bilaterally in subcortical regions of the brain, where they emit the electrical stimulation. They can now be placed almost anywhere in the brain and even on the surface just under the skull (extradural).

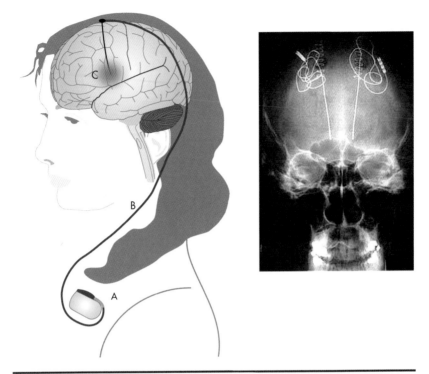

FIGURE 7-1. Deep brain stimulation.

The impulse generator **(A)**, the extension **(B)**, and the electrode implanted into subcortical regions of the brain **(C)**.

Source. X-ray image on the right provided by Helen Mayberg. Used with permission.

Typically, but not always, the neurosurgery to implant the device is performed under a combination of general and local anesthesia. The reason for local rather than generalized anesthesia is to allow the patient to participate in the proper placement of the electrode. For example, with essential tremor, the neurosurgeon wants to find the location that maximally quiets the tremors. However, with dystonia, which can take months to show benefits, the placement is done under general anesthesia. The electrode is simply placed in the best possible location.

The active portion of the probe actually contains four electrodes that can emit electrical signals. Figure 7–2 shows an example of a probe placed in the subthalamic nucleus as treatment for Parkinson's disease. The four sites on the lead of the probe can be

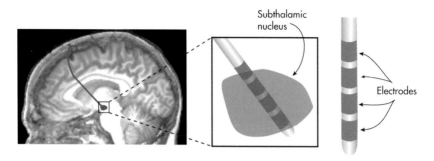

Subthalamic
nucleus

Electrodes

FIGURE 7–2. DBS electrode placed in the subthalamic nucleus to treat Parkinson's disease.
The lead of the probe has polyurethane insulation spaced around the four potential active electrode sites.

controlled to optimize the effect on the target site. An exciting new development is the use of leads that have many more sites, that allow for the ability to "steer" the current with more complicated electrical waveforms, or that are actually many small leads bundled together like a fork. The leads are getting more complicated, with the intention to provide a more beneficial pulse.

By adjusting which electrodes emit a signal, clinicians can mold the DBS effect. Figure 7–3 shows how activation of different electrodes in the probe changes the electrical signal, which in turn changes the parts of the brain stimulated and ultimately determines the effect of DBS on the patient.

There are a host of other variables that can be adjusted with DBS, not just which electrode emits a current. Voltage, pulse width, frequency, and bipolar or unipolar wave forms are just some of the other variables that can be adjusted. For example, a possible setting could be 3.5 volts, pulse width of 60, and a frequency of 130 Hz. Changing these variables can alter the benefits and side effects of the stimulation. Figuring out how to find the ideal stimulation setting in a given patient is a daunting task. With even only 4 electrodes, 10 different intensities, 3 pulse widths, and 5 different frequencies gives 600 different combinations ($4\times10\times3\times5=600$) for one side (multiply by 2 for bilateral implantation, which is common). Trying each one out for even 15 minutes could result in more than a week in the clinic and waiting room. Doctors are now experimenting with "intelligent" ways to explore which

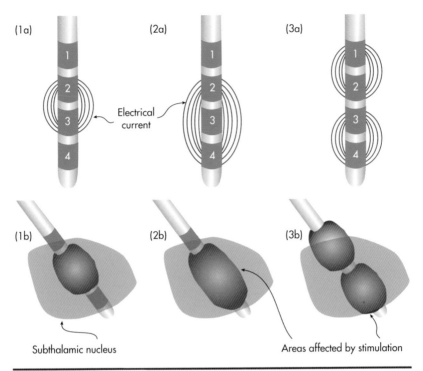

FIGURE 7-3. Electrical current production in DBS.

Electrical current can be produced from any two of the four electrodes. **(1a)** shows the current between electrodes 2 and 3. **(1b)** shows how much of the nucleus is stimulated with these settings. **(2a)** and **(2b)** are between electrodes 2 and 3. **(3a)** and **(3b)** are between electrodes 1 and 2 and between electrodes 3 and 4.

Source. Modified from Butson and McIntyre 2008.

parameters to use based on biomarkers, imaging, and even machine learning and artificial intelligence. It will only get more complicated as the technology improves, so solving this issue is important for the future of invasive DBS.

Responsive Neural Stimulation

Numerous alternative ways to directly stimulate the brain are continuously being explored. One can barely keep up with the new reports. Two techniques have risen to the top and are currently being studied. One is called *responsive neural stimulation* (RNS). This entails the addition of a microprocessor designed to sense

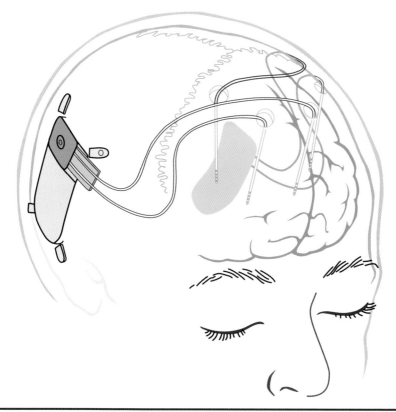

FIGURE 7–4. Responsive neural stimulation.

Bilateral impulse generators can detect abnormal electrical activity and respond with appropriate stimulation (patient's left side generator, behind the brain, is in *blue*). Electrodes can be placed deep into subcortical structures, as shown, or left superficially on the surface of the cortex (cortical brain stimulation).

the brain's electrical signals (through electroencephalography, or more accurately, electrocorticography) and deliver pulses when abnormal activity is detected (see Figure 7–4). This device is now approved for treatment-resistant epilepsy.

Cortical Brain Stimulation

Another promising technique is cortical brain stimulation. (This could almost be called "superficial" brain stimulation, in contrast to "deep" brain stimulation.) In this case, the electrodes are placed directly on the surface of the cortex. This is useful for problems that arise from disorders in the cortical gray matter, for example, when a seizure focus is in the cortex. To minimize infections and other side effects, the electrodes are placed below the skull but on top of the dura mater (see Figure 3–6 for reference).

What Does DBS Do to the Brain?

The mechanisms of DBS are incompletely understood (Kern and Kumar 2007). Regardless, the frequency of the stimulation is known to be important. Frequencies of greater than 100 Hz seem to be most effective, whereas frequencies of less than 50 Hz are of no benefit. The stimulation remains localized (about 2–3 mm), because the intensity of the current is small. The pulse width may determine the parts of the neuron that are affected. Longer pulse widths influence the cell body, while shorter pulse widths have more effect on the axons. These parameters (e.g., frequency, intensity, pulse width) can, of course, be modified to influence effects and side effects.

The ultimate effect of *constant* high-frequency DBS is reversible inhibition of the stimulated site. This is clear because the effects are similar to ablative surgery. Exactly how high-frequency stimulation "shuts down" the target site remains a mystery. Theories include

1. "Neuronal jamming" such that signals emitting from the site are incomprehensible and ineffective downstream.
2. Activation of inhibitory gamma-aminobutyric acid (GABA) neurons.
3. Stimulation of reciprocal inhibitory neurons.

Parkinson's Disease

The most common utilization of DBS is for treating medication-resistant Parkinson's disease. A brief review of the current understanding of Parkinson's disease provides a better understanding of how DBS affects the brain. The pathology of Parkinson's disease is centered on the basal ganglia (see Figure 7–5). The disease process starts with gradual destruction of the substantia nigra,

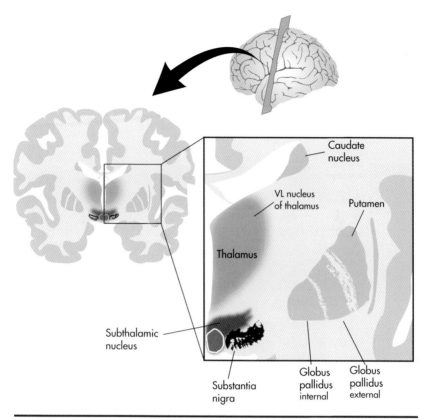

FIGURE 7–5. The basal ganglia.

The basal ganglia is made up of the caudate nucleus, putamen, subthalamic nucleus, and substantia nigra. VL=ventrolateral.

Source. Adapted from Bear et al. 2006.

which in turn has devastating effects on the other nuclei of the basal ganglia (Bear et al. 2006). This occurs subclinically without external symptoms, because the system has some reserve and is able to compensate for mild losses. (Actually, even before this, there is damage to the nucleus tractus solitarius. The astute reader will remember that this is where vagus nerve signals enter the body. That's right, researchers are now investigating using VNS to treat early Parkinson's disease.)

The downstream effect of a diminished signal coming out of the substantia nigra results in a stronger signal coming out of other nuclei. This has the paradoxical effect of putting the brakes

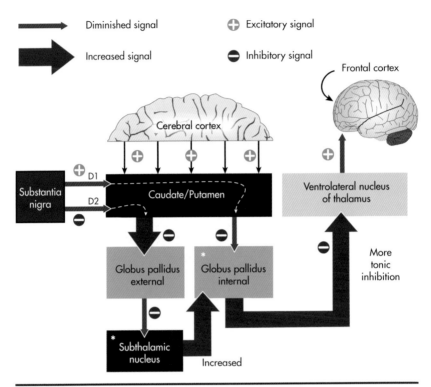

FIGURE 7–6. Signal enhancement and movement inhibition in Parkinson's disease.

Parkinson's disease starts with diminished output from the substantia nigra, which results in enhanced signals coming out of the subthalamic nucleus and globus pallidus interna. DBS electrode placement in either of these nuclei (*) reduces the inhibition on movement.

Source. Adapted from Purves et al. 2004.

on movement. Figure 7–6 outlines what many believe occurs in the basal ganglia with Parkinson's disease (Purves et al. 2004). Increased signals from the subthalamic nucleus and globus pallidus interna results in increased inhibition of the ventrolateral nucleus of the thalamus—which slows muscular movement.

The goal of most DBS for Parkinson's disease is to inhibit the enhanced inhibiting signals. In other words, high-frequency DBS (or ablative surgery) "releases the brakes," thus allowing movement to occur more normally. The two best locations for DBS for Parkinson's disease are the subthalamic nucleus and the globus pallidus interna. When these nuclei are inhibited with a DBS electrode, the brakes are removed and movement flows.

Beta Waves

Beta waves are an exciting area of research that hopes to make the DBS more responsive for Parkinson's disease. Basal ganglia cells sometimes emit an unusual rhythm called beta waves. Researchers are testing whether a closed-loop smart DBS device could detect those waves and then fire pulses that block them. This would be an intermittent-stimulation method rather than the continuous-stimulation method in current use. It would prolong the battery life and perhaps have a positive impact on the underlying neurodegenerative process.

Safety and Adverse Events

The most serious potential risk associated with DBS is from the neurosurgical procedure, particularly bleeding and stroke (Kern and Kumar 2007). This risk generally ranges from 1% to 3%. If a stroke occurs, it usually occurs during or within a few hours of surgery. Another risk is infection, which occurs in about 4%–5% of patients. If an infection occurs, it is usually not life threatening but may require immediate removal of the entire DBS system. It is important to realize that DBS, virtually alone among the brain stimulation treatments, has a small but nevertheless real risk of death (<1% depending on the location and type of electrodes). Because it requires repeated anesthesia, electroconvulsive therapy also has a theoretical risk of death, but the risk is only about 1 in 50,000 inductions.

DBS may lead to neuropsychiatric problems (Wichmann and Delong 2006). Some patients have developed paresthesias or involuntary movements. Other patients have developed cognitive side effects or mood changes that range from disinhibition, gambling, or, even worse, suicide. Most of these problems can be eliminated with adjustments to the stimulating parameters, but they are important to watch for.

Postmortem analysis of brains from patients with long-term DBS has revealed some subtle findings. Mild gliosis (the brain's inflammatory response) has been found around the electrode. Moderate cell loss proximal to the electrode tip has also been found.

Impulsive Behavior

The dopaminergic medications used to treat Parkinson's disease have been reported to increase impulsive behavior, such as pathological gambling (Dodd et al. 2005). A group at the University of Arizona initially demonstrated with a computer game that DBS will also increase impulsiveness (Frank et al. 2007). Their research suggests that the subthalamic nucleus sends a "hold your horses" signal to other parts of the brain to allow more time to weigh attractive choices. The DBS patients were quicker to rush their choices when their stimulators were on, temporarily blocking the subthalamic nucleus brakes.

Critical Review of Randomized Controlled Trials of DBS in Neuropsychiatric Applications

Parkinson's Disease

The medications for Parkinson's disease are generally effective but problematic. As the disease progresses, medications lose their effectiveness in most patients. Thus, patients receiving long-term treatment struggle with three phases of response through any day:

1. "On": moving easily
2. "Off": stiff, difficult movement
3. "On" with dyskinesias—involuntary movements similar to tics or chorea

DBS is a viable alternative for patients with drug-induced motor fluctuations or those with intractable tremor (Wichmann and Delong 2006). The best candidates are patients who respond to levodopa and are free of dementia or psychiatric disorders. Choosing the right time to implant a device is part of the clinical challenge.

The pivotal trials testing for DBS with Parkinson's disease were conducted at 18 centers in the late 1990s (Obeso et al. 2001). Although no patients received a sham implantation, double-blind assessments were conducted at 6 months by assessing motor function with the stimulator "on" and again when "off."

Two sites for implantation were used in the original studies: subthalamic nuclei and the globus pallidus interna. The subthalamic nucleus has become the preferred site for most surgeons. Figure 7–7 shows unblinded assessments of motor function before and after and with and without medication. Likewise, patient diaries of waking hours in "on," "off," or dyskinesias are included. Note that the DBS does not significantly improve the motor score compared to medications alone but does improve the amount of time patients spend with good mobility.

Since the publication of the pivotal studies, further research continues to support benefits from DBS for the movement disorders associated with Parkinson's disease. A 5-year follow-up of the first 49 patients to receive bilateral stimulation of the subthalamic nucleus found continued improvement in motor function (Krack et al. 2003). A meta-analysis of 45 studies concluded that motor function improved by 54% in patients with subthalamic nucleus stimulation and 40% in patients with globus pallidus interna stimulation (Weaver et al. 2005).

Later, a randomized study compared DBS with medical management in 37 Parkinson's disease patients (Deuschl et al. 2006).

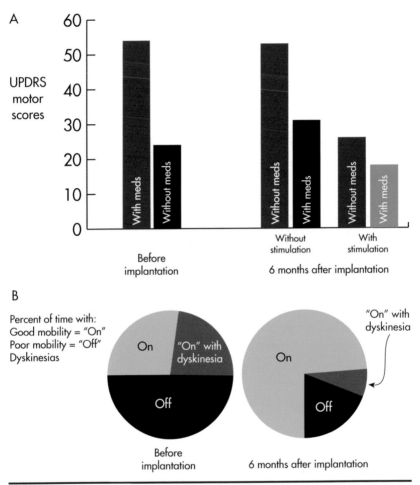

FIGURE 7–7. Patient responses to DBS placed in the subthalamic nucleus.

(A) Unified Parkinson's Disease Rating Scale (UPDRS) motor scores before and after implantation, with and without medications. **(B)** Patient diaries before and after implantation, reporting percentage of time in each state of mobility.

Source. Adapted from Obeso et al. 2001.

The authors reported superior motor function as well as improved quality of life for the patients receiving stimulation and medication compared with medication only. This study also provided a better assessment of adverse events. Although the patients receiving just medications experienced greater overall frequency of side effects (64% vs. 50%), the patients with DBS had a greater incidence of serious adverse events (13% vs. 4%), including one death from intracerebral hemorrhage. Psychiatric sequalae were common.

Finally, it is important to remember that DBS only improves motor function. The natural progression of akinesia, postural instability, and cognitive function are unaffected by DBS.

Listening for the Right Spot

Modern neurosurgeons use imaging scans and knowledge of the neuroanatomy to place the electrode tip in the precise location. However, they also use the sound of the neuronal activity to help guide them. The electrode captures cell activity during placement. The sound can be amplified and played for the surgeon in the operating room. Experienced surgeons recognize the "sounds" of different tissue and use that to help them find the right spot.

Tremor

The treatment of tremors was actually the first use of DBS and continues to be a major application of the device (Wichmann and Delong 2006). Essential tremor is the most common cause of tremor, but there are several other kinds of tremors that respond to DBS: brain stem (Holmes) tremor and tremors associated with Parkinson's disease or multiple sclerosis. The ventral intermediate nucleus of the thalamus (Vim) is the usual site for placement of the DBS electrodes. The stimulation of the Vim appears to be effective for most forms of tremor regardless of the etiology.

The pivotal trials of DBS for parkinsonian or essential tremor were conducted in Europe at 13 neurosurgical centers (Limousin et al. 1999). One hundred and eleven patients received implants, and the results were reported at the 12-month follow-up. Upper and lower limb tremors were significantly reduced in 85% of the patients. Postural tremors were reduced in 89%.

Numerous other subsequent studies continue to demonstrate beneficial effects for essential tremor with DBS (Wichmann and Delong 2006). Specifically, the procedure improves quality of life, and the benefits persist. However, one small follow-up study with DBS found tolerance developing in some patients with essential tremor.

Figure 7–8 shows some perplexing results from functional imaging studies conducted on 10 patients with DBS for essential tremor (Perlmutter et al. 2002). Patients were scanned with the stimulator "on" and "off," and the results were averaged for the group. Areas of increased blood flow during stimulation are shown in color. Note that the stimulation actually increases blood flow to the thalamus (where the electrodes are placed) and to the supplementary motor area.

These results were not expected because DBS of the Vim seems to have the same effect as ablation. How can removing the Vim and increasing the activity of the Vim (as shown with increased blood flow) have the same effect? These results accentuate the limited understanding we have of what DBS is doing to the brain and the relationship between blood flow and regional activity.

Dystonia

Dystonia is characterized by twisting, repetitive movements or abnormal postures caused by irregular muscle contractions (Wichmann and Delong 2006). Dystonia can be primary (inherited or birth related) or secondary (such as caused by neuropsychiatric medications). Dystonia is classified into two forms: generalized and focal. The focal form can usually be managed with botulinum toxin injections, but the generalized form is less responsive to medications. Some patients are almost completely incapacitated with the movements.

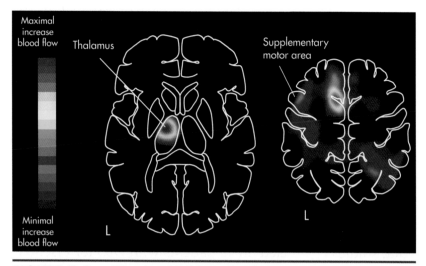

FIGURE 7–8.   Effects of DBS on the brain.

Positron emission tomography scans on patients with DBS for essential tremor. The color shows areas of increased blood flow during times of stimulation.

Source.   Adapted from Perlmutter et al. 2002.

Earlier work involving ablation of either the globus pallidus interna or the thalamus led others to try DNS for dystonia. The globus pallidus interna has become the most common site of stimulation. Pivotal trials were never conducted because it was believed the eventual market demand in dystonia was insufficient to justify industry funding such a study. However, remarkable individual responses with DBS led the FDA to grant approval on a "compassionate use" basis. For example, patient Kari Weiner had been afflicted with dystonia for 7 years and confined to a wheelchair by the age of 13 (Horgan 2005). Now, with DBS, she walks without assistance. The interested reader can search "Kari Weiner" and "dystonia" or locate the reference to find more details about her case.

A randomized European study of 40 patients with primary segmental or generalized dystonia was conducted (Kupsch et al. 2006). Half the patients had the stimulation started immediately, whereas the other half had initiation of stimulation delayed by 3 months. At 3 months, patients were blindly rated on the basis of video examinations and compared with baseline. Patients who received stimulation had significant improvements in movement scores (39%) and disability (38%). Patients in the sham arm had small, nonsignificant improvements.

Chronic Pain

There is a long history of neurosurgical interventions to relieve chronic pain. It is intuitively appealing to sever the connection between the offending site and the area that perceives the pain in the brain. Unfortunately, it is not that straightforward. The results are often temporary, and symptoms frequently return. Brain stimulation offers a way to adapt the treatment to match the dynamic and evolving nature of the pain condition. The frequency, pulse width, and intensity of stimulation can be altered as the pathology changes.

Treatment of pain may have been the first use for brain stimulation (see Figure 1–2 in Chapter 1). DBS for chronic pain has been studied sporadically for over 50 years, although only in the past 20 years have we had the technology for continuous stimulation (Kringelbach et al. 2007). There are numerous small studies following the effects of stimulation of various regions for various different forms of pain. In general, it is believed that stimulation of the periventricular/periaqueductal gray matter is best for nociceptive pain, while stimulation of the sensory thalamic nuclei is best for neuropathic pain (Kern and Kumar 2007). The reports look encouraging. However, as with the ablation studies, it is not so straightforward.

In the 1990s, Medtronics (the manufacturer of the DBS device) conducted two multicenter trials of DBS for chronic pain at the same time it was conducting studies for Parkinson's disease and essential tremor (Coffey 2001). The results of the pain studies were disappointing (high dropout rate and poor efficacy), and the manufacturer abandoned the studies and did not apply for FDA approval. A definitive large, randomized multicenter trial establishing sufficient efficacy has not yet been conducted.

Another option for chronic pain entails stimulation of the motor cortex. In this procedure the electrodes are placed directly on the dura mater over the motor cortex where the pain is located. This use is not FDA approved but is relatively common (Birknes et al. 2006). At our institution (MUSC), the neurosurgeon asks for a transcranial magnetic stimulation (TMS) evaluation of the motor cortex prior to surgery to have a better understanding of the location of the desired section of the motor cortex.

Epilepsy

The best treatment for chronic epilepsy is actually resective brain surgery of the area of the brain where the seizure starts—a surgery William Penfield was doing in the 1930s (see Chapter 1). Most seizures arise in the medial temporal lobe, which controls language. Thus, many patients cannot have their seizure focus removed because they may become mute. NeuroPace conducted a large clinical trial in these patients using their responsive stimulation device, a device that learns, through trial and error with each seizure, how to identify the prodrome of the seizure and inhibit this before it gets in full swing (see Figure 7–4).

Depression

The use of DBS in patients with treatment-resistant depression was widely reported in the lay press. Unfortunately, two large clinical trials were dramatically disappointing. While DBS was potentially an exciting new option for depressed patients who fail all other therapies, the clinical trials have failed and the enthusiasm has waned. To make matters even more confusing, the different groups used different technologies while also stimulating different sites in the brain—the subgenual cingulate and the anterior limb of the internal capsule, nucleus accumbens (ALICNA).

Subgenual cingulate. The most widely cited studies have been by Helen Mayberg and her group in Toronto (Mayberg et al. 2005). Mayberg conceptualizes depression as a systems disorder. That is, the network modulating mood gets out of sync in patients with depression. It had been noted that patients with depression showed greater activity in the subgenual cingulate cortex, or what is also called Brodmann area 25, compared with control subjects (George et al. 1997; Wu et al. 1992). Research by a different group replicated and extended these insights (Greicius et al. 2007) (see Figure 7–9).

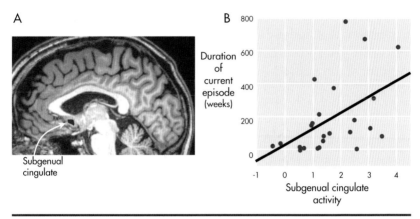

FIGURE 7-9. Subgenual cingulate activity and depression.
Activity in the subgenual cingulate **(A)** correlates with duration of the
current episode of depression **(B)**.
Source. Adapted from Greicius et al. 2007.

In this study, the resting activity in the subgenual cingulate correlated with the duration of the episode of depression. Other research has shown that patients with depression who respond to
treatment show a decrease in activity in the subgenual cingulate
(Wu et al. 1992).

With this background, the Toronto group implanted bilateral
electrodes in six patients with treatment-resistant depression. (Actually, the electrodes were placed in the white matter tracts next to
the subgenual cingulate because that location of the cingulate is
hard to reach.) Remarkably, all patients spontaneously reported in
the operating room acute positive effects with stimulation such as
a "sudden calmness" or "disappearance of the void." At 6 months,
four of the six patients still had good responses to the stimulation
(symptoms cut in half), but very few were totally free of symptoms (remission). Positron emission tomography scans of the responders showed decreased activity in the subgenual cingulate.
These positive results have spurred further studies, including a
large randomized controlled trial conducted by Boston Scientific.
The FDA required interim analyses of the trial in order to minimize
harm to patients. The trial was stopped prematurely because there
was no difference between those patients implanted with the DBS
turned on and those implanted with the DBS not yet turned on.
Both groups had similar response rates.

> ## Patenting the Brain?
>
> One of the more interesting (and troubling) developments spinning off DBS research is that several scientists are patenting regions of the brain for therapeutic stimulation. Whether or not these patents are legally permissible, we worry this is not a good development for advancement of the field.

ALICNA (anterior limb of the internal capsule, nucleus accumbens). This acronym is a complex attempt to describe a region of the brain that was initially used in depression, pain, or OCD neurosurgeries. A different multisite group implanted the electrodes in a manner that interrupts the white matter tracts connecting the cingulate to the orbitofrontal cortex. The tip of these electrodes abuts on the nucleus accumbens. The FDA calls this approach ALICNA (anterior limb of the internal capsule, nucleus accumbens). In an initial study of 15 patients with treatment-resistant depression, in which DBS was added to stable background medication, this multisite group found that about half of the patients had responded by 6 and 12 months, with less than a third achieving remission (Dougherty et al. 2007). Although there was some worsening of suicidal thoughts, there were no suicide attempts.

Medtronic then conducted a large trial in which depressed patients received implants at this site. The results were unfortunately the same as for the subgenual cingulate approach. The study was halted prematurely because of a failure to find a difference between active and sham.

What went wrong with these DBS depression studies? The initial cases seemed so promising, with patients reporting astounding recoveries in the operating room when the device was first turned "on." Yet controlled trials failed to show a difference between real and sham stimulation. Part of the problem is the age-old pattern of publicizing the best individual cases. Another problem may be the design of the studies. Everyone received a lot of attention, and everyone, on average, improved by 30%—and these were supposedly patients with treatment-resistant depression.

Clearly the placebo arm included something therapeutic—another age-old problem in mental health treatment. Finally, we conceptualize depression as a network disorder, not a localized dysfunction emanating from one critical group of neurons. Consequently, stimulating one small area of the brain seems insufficient. Psychiatric disorders, unlike some neurological disorders, involve wide networks of the brain. However, interest remains and more studies are being planned. Stay tuned.

Nucleus accumbens, median forebrain bundle. Schlaepfer and his group in Germany have experimented with stimulating the nucleus accumbens—what is sometimes called the brain's pleasure center (Schlaepfer et al. 2008). They postulated that activity in the nucleus accumbens is insufficient in depressed patients, which may explain the anhedonia and lack of motivation these patients experience. Schlaepfer's group implanted DBS electrodes in three patients with extremely resistant forms of depression. They reported that clinical ratings improved for all three patients when the stimulator was on and worsened when it was turned off. They have since moved the location of the electrodes to the white matter fibers leading into this region, called the median forebrain bundle. These small open studies are promising. A double-blind study at this site has not been performed. We hope that it would have a different result for depression than did the other two sites.

The nucleus accumbens work is of particular interest because of its similarities to the work Heath was conducting in the 1950s and 1960s (see "Emotional Pacemaker" in Chapter 1). Heath also implanted stimulating devices to enhance pleasure in depressed patients. Ultimately, he found the benefits dissipated with time. It will be important to establish whether modern DBS has any enduring efficacy for depression.

Obsessive-Compulsive Disorder

In the past, for patients with severe, unremitting OCD, ablative neurosurgery has been an option. Small lesions of the anterior capsule or anterior cingulate have been effective in about a third of the patients. DBS offers the option of interrupting the obsessive circuitry without destroying tissue. Greenberg et al. (2006) initially published a promising open-label study. They followed eight patients for 36 months after implantation. They reported that four patients had improvements of greater than 35% on the OCD scale, while an additional two patients had improvements of more than 25%. More recently, the National Institutes of Health conducted a large, randomized clinical trial of DBS for OCD.

The OCD/DBS study did not go as anticipated. It was difficult to find qualified patients who were interested. They had to extend the length of the trial, and in the end, it lasted 10 years with only 18 patients receiving implants. Active treatment received stimulation immediately after the surgery, while the sham group waited 6 months before the device was turned on. At the conclusion of this long, drawn-out study, the active-treatment group was not statistically improved as measured by the primary outcome—the Yale-Brown Obsessive Compulsive Scale. However, ratings for two measures of functional assessment were superior in the active treatment.

These mixed results are a disappointment and, as with the depression studies, enthusiasm has dwindled.

A Word of Caution

It is important to remember that Freeman and Watts (1950), in their initial glowing assessment of the frontal lobotomy, reported that out of 711 lobotomies, 45% yielded good results and an additional 33% yielded fair results. Later studies found far more minimal effects, with major side effects. This stresses the importance of having outcome assessments conducted by independent observers and proceeding cautiously with new invasive technology. The recent failed DBS studies in depression and OCD also highlight the need for caution and rigorous science before accepting new brain stimulation methods, especially those that are expensive and have potentially severe side effects.

Summary of Clinical Use

DBS is FDA-approved and effective for treatment-resistant Parkinson's disease and is also used for dystonia, essential tremor, epilepsy, and OCD. Cortical stimulation over motor cortex has been used for many years by neurosurgeons for intractable pain. The recent randomized trials of DBS for depression or OCD have not separated active stimulation from zero stimulation. In summary, DBS is effective for four neurological conditions but has yet to show effectiveness for a psychiatric disorder.

For all disorders potentially treated with DBS, it is important to know if the effects seen are DBS related or are caused by the insertion effect of the microtrauma of passing the wire. Given the history of the over-rapid adoption of frontal lobotomies, it is important to proceed cautiously with DBS for other conditions, because there is potential morbidity and even mortality.

References

Bear MF, Connors BW, Paradiso MA: Neuroscience: Exploring the Brain. Baltimore, MD, Lippincott Williams & Wilkins, 2006

Benabid AL, Pollak P, Seigneuret E, et al: Chronic VIM thalamic stimulation in Parkinson's disease, essential tremor and extra-pyramidal dyskinesias. Acta Neurochir Suppl (Wien) 58(suppl):39–44, 1993 8109299

Birknes JK, Sharan A, Rezai AR: Treatment of chronic pain with neurostimulation. Prog Neurol Surg 19:197–207, 2006 17033155

Butson CR, McIntyre CC: Current steering to control the volume of tissue activated during deep brain stimulation. Brain Stimul 1:7–15, 2008 19142235

Coffey RJ: Deep brain stimulation for chronic pain: results of two multicenter trials and a structured review. Pain Med 2(3):183–192, 2001 15102250

Deuschl G, Schade-Brittinger C, Krack P, et al: A randomized trial of deep-brain stimulation for Parkinson's disease. N Engl J Med 355(9):896–908, 2006 16943402

Dodd ML, Klos KJ, Bower JH, et al: Pathological gambling caused by drugs used to treat Parkinson disease. Arch Neurol 62(9):1377–1381, 2005 16009751

Dougherty DD, Malone D, Carpenter L, et al: Long-Term Outcomes of Ventral Capsule/Ventral Striatum DBS for Highly Treatment-Resistant Depression. Boca Raton, FL, American College of Psychopharmacology, 2007

Frank MJ, Samanta J, Moustafa AA, et al: Hold your horses: impulsivity, deep brain stimulation, and medication in parkinsonism. Science 318(5854):1309–1312, 2007 17962524

Freeman W, Watts JW: Psychosurgery in the Treatment of Mental Disorder and Intractable Pain, 2nd Edition. Springfield, IL, Charles C Thomas, 1950

George MS, Ketter TA, Parekh PI, et al: Blunted left cingulate activation in mood disorder subjects during a response interference task (the Stroop). J Neuropsychiatry Clin Neurosci 9(1):55–63, 1997 9017529

Greenberg BD, Malone DA, Friehs GM, et al: Three-year outcomes in deep brain stimulation for highly resistant obsessive-compulsive disorder. Neuropsychopharmacology 31(11):2384–2393, 2006 16855529

Greicius MD, Flores BH, Menon V, et al: Resting-state functional connectivity in major depression: abnormally increased contributions from subgenual cingulate cortex and thalamus. Biol Psychiatry 62(5):429–437, 2007 17210143

Horgan J: The forgotten era of brain chips. Sci Am 293(4):66–73, 2005 16196255

Kern DS, Kumar R: Deep brain stimulation. Neurologist 13(5):237–252, 2007 17848864

Krack P, Batir A, Van Blercom N, et al: Five-year follow-up of bilateral stimulation of the subthalamic nucleus in advanced Parkinson's disease. N Engl J Med 349(20):1925–1934, 2003 14614167

Kringelbach ML, Jenkinson N, Owen SLF, et al: Translational principles of deep brain stimulation. Nat Rev Neurosci 8(8):623–635, 2007 17637800

Kupsch A, Benecke R, Müller J, et al: Pallidal deep-brain stimulation in primary generalized or segmental dystonia. N Engl J Med 355(19):1978–1990, 2006 17093249

Limousin P, Speelman JD, Gielen F, et al: Multicentre European study of thalamic stimulation in parkinsonian and essential tremor. J Neurol Neurosurg Psychiatry 66(3):289–296, 1999 10084526

Mayberg HS, Lozano AM, Voon V, et al: Deep brain stimulation for treatment-resistant depression. Neuron 45(5):651–660, 2005 15748841

Nicholls M: Pioneers of cardiology: Rune Elmqvist, MD. Circulation 115(22):f109–f111, 2007 17548737

Obeso JA, Olanow CW, Rodriguez-Oroz MC, et al: Deep-brain stimulation of the subthalamic nucleus or the pars interna of the globus pallidus in Parkinson's disease. N Engl J Med 345(13):956–963, 2001 11575287

Perlmutter JS, Mink JW, Bastian AJ, et al: Blood flow responses to deep brain stimulation of thalamus. Neurology 58(9):1388–1394, 2002 12011286

Purves D, Augustine GJ, Fitzpatrick D, et al: Neuroscience, 3rd Edition. Sunderland, MA, Sinauer, 2004

Schlaepfer TE, Cohen MX, Frick C, et al: Deep brain stimulation to reward circuitry alleviates anhedonia in refractory major depression. Neuropsychopharmacology 33(2):368–377, 2008 17429407

Spangler WJ, Cosgrove GR, Ballantine HT Jr, et al: Magnetic resonance image-guided stereotactic cingulotomy for intractable psychiatric disease. Neurosurgery 38(6):1071–1076, discussion 1076–1078, 1996 8727135

Weaver F, Follett K, Hur K, et al: Deep brain stimulation in Parkinson disease: a metaanalysis of patient outcomes. J Neurosurg 103(6):956–967, 2005 16381181

Wichmann T, Delong MR: Deep brain stimulation for neurologic and neuropsychiatric disorders. Neuron 52(1):197–204, 2006 17015236

Wu JC, Gillin JC, Buchsbaum MS, et al: Effect of sleep deprivation on brain metabolism of depressed patients. Am J Psychiatry 149(4):538–543, 1992 1554042

CHAPTER 8

Transcranial Direct Current Stimulation

Introduction and History

Transcranial direct current stimulation (tDCS) is perhaps one of the simplest ways of focally stimulating the brain. Similar techniques were practiced almost immediately after electricity was "discovered" in the 1800s. Passing a direct current through muscle, or the brain, was in vogue in Europe. For example, one of Charcot's residents, Georges Duchenne de Boulogne, traveled around Paris with a small generator and battery and passed electricity through patients' muscles, examining the effects on numerous disorders and using it to better understand muscle-nerve innervations, particularly in the muscular dystrophies (see Figure 8–1) (George 1994). Others began applying direct current through the brain. Because of the lack of benefits, this approach was largely dropped as a treatment in Europe and the United States.

However, tDCS continued to be studied and used in Russia during the 1940s up until the present time. tDCS is inexpensive and easy to use, which may have enhanced its appeal to the Soviet Socialists. It was sometimes called "electrosleep therapy" because patients would sometimes nap or sleep during the 30-minute treatments (Gomez and Mikhail 1979). Most of the tDCS done in Russia was not delivered in clinical trials and was largely anecdotally used for the treatment of alcoholism, pain, depression, or a combination of these (Feighner et al. 1973).

Dr. Walter Paulus and his group in Göttingen, Germany, led a resurrection of this technology, and there is now active investigation of tDCS throughout the world, with several thousand articles in peer-reviewed journals. Clearly, tDCS has an effect on the brain—it can boost cortical excitability and improve memory in healthy people. Whether these effects can be used therapeutically remains to be determined, and there is no U.S. Food and Drug Administration (FDA)–approved indication. Fortunately, there is at least one positive randomized controlled trial with tDCS in poststroke aphasia, which is discussed later (Fridriksson et al. 2018a, 2018b).

How Is It Done?

Quite simply, tDCS involves passing a weak (usually 1- to 4-milliampere) direct current through the brain between two electrodes. The current enters the brain from the anode, travels through the tissue, and exits out the cathode (see Figure 8–2). Some researchers refer to this as either *cathodal tDCS* or *anodal tDCS*, depending on which electrode is placed over the region that is being modified.

The administration of tDCS is relatively easy. Many researchers simply use damp sponges as the electrodes. These can be placed anywhere on the scalp inside a nonconducting holder and are held in place with an elastic headband.

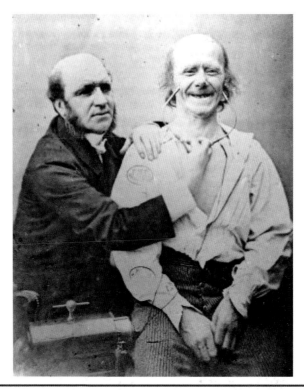

FIGURE 8–1.   An early form of "something like tDCS."
Duchenne de Boulogne passed direct current through the muscles of
the face and stimulated the muscles involved in smiling. Duchenne
wrote about the differences between a "false" and a "true" smile. Because he stimulated muscles and not the brain or nervous tissue,
Duchenne's work is not technically tDCS.

What Does tDCS Do to the Brain?

Exactly what happens to the brain with tDCS remains unknown
despite a great deal of research. However, experiments with animals, humans, and even direct recordings from individual neurons give a general idea. Starting with the basics, the anode (which
is negative; remember A-N, AN) is where electrons enter the brain.
The cathode (which is positive) is where the electricity exits the
brain. Thus, there is a buildup of negative charge under the exiting
cathode as the electrons line up to get on the exiting electrode (like
passengers waiting to get on the subway, bunching at the door).

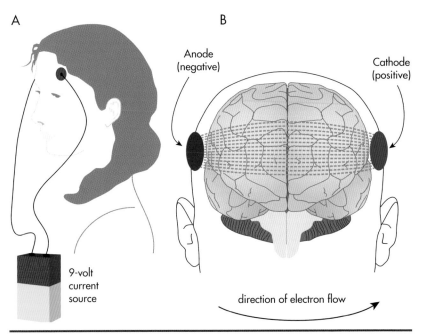

FIGURE 8-2. Transcranial direct current stimulation.

The tDCS device encompasses attaching an anode and cathode from an energy source generating direct current **(A)**. The passage of current through the brain induces changes that are believed to be therapeutic **(B)**.

A smaller cathode can produce a more focal delivery of charge to a brain region, as more charge lines up right below the exit door. Thus, you can shape or influence the size of the brain region being affected by changing the size of the cathodal electrode (smaller size is more focused) or changing the size and location of the anodal electrode (Nitsche et al. 2007).

The behavioral effects of what happens under the exiting cathode are not as simple as one would hope. In most studies the area under the anode is more active (or excited) and the area under the cathode is more inhibited. For example, stimulation of the motor regions produces such results, and this is being exploited as a possible treatment for stroke.

However, the brain is enormously complex, and there are studies in which the brain region under the anode is behaviorally *inhibited.* For example, in one study examining the latency of a visual evoked response, 10 minutes of anodal tDCS reduced visual evoked potential amplitudes, while 10 minutes of cathodal tDCS increased amplitudes for several minutes following stimulation (Accornero et al. 2007). Thus, in this study there was behavioral inhibition under the anode and excitation under the cathode. It appears that the different regions of the brain with different morphology, layering, and cellular composition can have different responses to direct current stimulation (Rahman et al. 2013).

tDCS Compared With ECT

tDCS uses small currents over 20–30 minutes. It is constant, and the brain has time to accommodate to the gentle current. By contrast, electroconvulsive therapy (ECT) uses a short, powerful, bidirectional current, which typically has a waveform that makes it resemble an alternating current. The brain cannot adapt to the ECT stimulus, and a seizure is induced. However, the total amount of electricity used in a session of ECT compared with a session of tDCS is not that different. Importantly, the brain reacts differently because of the different type of the stimulus and the very different time domains of application.

The human head is a poor conductor of electricity. tDCS, like ECT, is extremely inefficient at stimulating the brain, because at least 50% of the current is lost to the surrounding tissue. That is why you can use much less electricity when you bypass the skull and touch neurons directly as you do with deep brain stimulation or with transcranial magnetic stimulation (TMS; in which the magnetic field passes through the skull).

Finally, as with all stimulation techniques, the ability to induce enduring effects beyond the time of administration is essential for practical clinical applications. With tDCS, it appears that the focal and behavioral changes can persist after the electrodes are removed. In studies of tDCS on motor cortex, for example, tDCS-induced inhibition or excitation can last for several minutes to an hour or so. The improvements seen in the tDCS poststroke aphasia study lasted for several weeks—an encouraging finding. Whether therapeutic changes can endure for weeks or months with tDCS and in other disorders remains to be determined.

tDCS, tACS, and tRNS

The language and acronyms get a bit confusing. Theoretically, one could send electrical signals in an alternating current pattern, but unidirectionally (unipolar, not bipolar pulses). Then, electrical charge would distribute asymmetrically between the cathode and anode. This idea is called *transcranial alternating current stimulation* (tACS). As with many of the stimulation methods, you could massively increase the current and use this to create a powerful focal seizure. This has, in fact, been done in primates. We call this method "seizure producing tACS" (see Figure 8–3). Others, including the pioneers of this method, refer to this as *focal electrically applied seizure therapy* (FEAST)—a topic discussed in Chapter 4, "Electroconvulsive Therapy." One can also simultaneously stimulate with a range of different frequencies. This is called *transcranial random noise stimulation* (tRNS; Mulquiney et al. 2011).

Safety and Adverse Events

Side effects of tDCS depend on the placement of the electrode, whether it is anodal or cathodal, the intensity of the stimulation, and the length of time the patient is treated. Skin burns can occur, and some patients feel uncomfortable or have reported dizziness. Modern treatments are minimally troublesome at worst (Antal et al. 2017).

Paulus and colleagues reported their results in 567 patients and subjects who had received tDCS in challenge studies over the motor, parietal, or occipital cortex (Poreisz et al. 2007). Remarkably, none of the patients requested that the stimulation be terminated. About 70% of subjects noticed a mild tingling sensation under the electrode. One-third of subjects felt fatigue after treatment, and one-third also felt "itching" under the electrode. Headache (11%), nausea (3%), and insomnia (1%) were also found but less frequently.

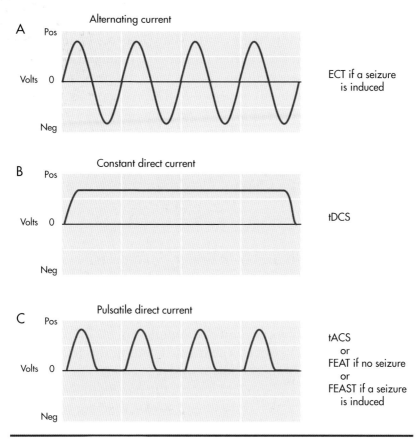

FIGURE 8–3. Waveforms for different techniques.

Different ways of delivering electrical current (and whether or not a seizure is induced) have different names in the literature. ECT=electroconvulsive therapy; FEAST= focal electrically applied seizure therapy; FEAT=focal electrically applied therapy; tACS = transcranial alternating current stimulation; tDCS=transcranial direct current stimulation.

Critical Review of Randomized Controlled Trials of tDCS in Neuropsychiatric Applications

Many studies with tDCS have focused on healing the sick. However, the vast majority of tDCS research has dealt with performance enhancement in healthy subjects. For example, video gamers, athletes, and college students are using tDCS to improve their scores and reduce their times. Many impressive testimonials can be found on the internet (although we remain skeptical). It is beyond the scope of this book to review the performance enhancement studies, but it is clear that tDCS can focally excite or inhibit the brain. This impressive and growing body of research convinces us that there are perhaps clinical uses of tDCS yet to be discovered. This is why we have given tDCS a standalone chapter despite there being no clear clinical indication or FDA approval for tDCS (Brunoni et al. 2012).

Stroke

Numerous small studies with healthy volunteers have shown that tDCS can enhance motor function and control. The next logical step is to apply the technique to patients whose motor control has been damaged because of a stroke. The unique qualities of tDCS offer possibilities beyond just stimulating the damaged tissue. Some research suggests that constraining the unaffected, healthy side of the brain actually improves healing. For example, constraining the good arm and forcing the patient to use the impaired arm improves recovery after a stroke affecting the upper limb. This is called *constraint induced movement therapy* (Liepert 2006).

Theoretically, tDCS could be able to mimic this therapeutic process. That is, one could excite the damaged side while inhibiting the healthy side. When the anode is placed over the injury, it should excite the neurons beneath it. Likewise, if the cathode is placed over the healthy side, it should provide some inhibition of those neurons. In summary, however, the work in motor stroke is still preliminary without large clear effects in well-conducted, sham-controlled trials (Alonso-Alonso et al. 2007; Fregni and Pascual-Leone 2007).

Recently, Julius Fridriksson, working with one of us (M.S.G.), completed perhaps the most promising study to date with tDCS and stroke. Seventy-four stroke patients with long-term (>6 months) aphasia were enrolled and randomly assigned to receive active or sham tDCS for 3 weeks (15 sessions, 30 minutes each). Importantly, the tDCS or sham was applied at the same time that patients were completing a computerized speech therapy naming program. Patients who received active tDCS could name 13 more words after the 3 weeks, compared with only 8 new words in those who received sham. This study was statistically significant both in a futility analysis (i.e., "Should we just stop this line of work?") and in a more conventional efficacy analysis (Fridriksson et al. 2018b). Quite interestingly, the patients with a certain genetic variant of brain-derived neurotrophic factor were those who improved most. tDCS is thus likely promoting plasticity in the brain during the speech therapy and is doing it to a greater degree in those who are genetically more prone to brain plasticity (Fridriksson et al. 2018a). Is five more words, or a 70% increase compared with the control subjects, really clinically meaningful? Well, let's put it this way: Neither of us has strapped a 9-volt battery to our heads to improve the writing of this book (although some have suggested we should). Yet we both agree that if we were to have a stroke and could not talk, we would want tDCS during our speech therapy.

Future Possibilities

As with all of the new stimulation techniques, there have been groups trying out the technology in almost all neuropsychiatric disorders. Single-site, small-sample studies have suggested some positive effects of tDCS in pain, migraine, fibromyalgia, depression, and epilepsy, to name a few. Overall, the results have been disappointing. Perhaps the most work has been conducted in tinnitus, depression, and epilepsy. We examine these each in some detail.

Pain

TMS has proven to have analgesic effects (see Figure 6–7). Why not tDCS? Jeff Borckardt and others have completed a series of postoperative studies in which the tDCS is applied over the sensory representation that has been affected or operated on, immediately following surgery. This approach has shown effects with postsurgical knee or gastric surgery (Borckardt et al. 2017; Glaser et al. 2016). At a time when everyone is looking for nonopiate approaches to pain management, we are disappointed that a manufacturer has not pursued FDA approval for this treatment. There are also small trials suggesting some use of tDCS for chronic pain, although none of these studies are of the highest quality, and this use is not FDA approved (Castillo-Saavedra et al. 2016).

Tinnitus

There is no treatment for tinnitus. tDCS seemed like an option and showed some promise in small studies. The larger, controlled studies have been disappointing, with positive results found only during a brief time after treatment—and no better than sham control (Landgrebe et al. 2017).

Depression

Finally, after a long delay, several large international studies using tDCS to treat depression have been completed. Unfortunately, they have been disappointing as well. It appears that if tDCS does work in depression (or other disorders), it needs to be combined with some other active treatment. Thus, tDCS might function as a catalyst; something that enhances the benefits of the primary treatment, such as psychotherapy.

Do-It-Yourself and Home Use of tDCS

Perhaps because tDCS is so inexpensive, and it cannot cause a seizure in the way that rTMS might, there is a very large industry selling tDCS devices for a variety of unsubstantiated conditions and claims (Bikson et al. 2018). Some companies suggest that tDCS can change someone's mood, and they offer calming and stimulating forms of tDCS. Others claim, without published data, that tDCS can improve motor or cognitive skills. While we wish this were true, the reality is that there are no definitive studies showing that tDCS can make you smarter, faster, or quicker in a general way. Although some studies have found improvement on a specific task (Scheldrup et al. 2014), it does not generalize to any other test or function, and the effects do not persist.

Summary of Clinical Use

Transcranial direct current stimulation is an exciting new tool that offers an inexpensive brain stimulation device that can be safely used at home. Unfortunately, there are few clinically useful applications as of this writing. The recent poststroke aphasia study has the strongest scientific evidence and stands alone as a beacon in the forest of disappointing studies. tDCS, like many of the stimulation techniques, followed the pattern of discovery, overuse, misuse, and then a reawakening with more modern approaches. tDCS likely will be useful in the future, especially when coupled with pharmacological and behavioral approaches to reshape circuit behavior in health or disease.

References

Accornero N, Li Voti P, La Riccia M, et al: Visual evoked potentials modulation during direct current cortical polarization. Exp Brain Res 178(2):261–266, 2007 17051377

Alonso-Alonso M, Fregni F, Pascual-Leone A: Brain stimulation in poststroke rehabilitation. Cerebrovasc Dis 24(suppl 1):157–166, 2007 17971652

Antal A, Alekseichuk I, Bikson M, et al: Low intensity transcranial electric stimulation: safety, ethical, legal regulatory and application guidelines. Clin Neurophysiol 128(9):1774–1809, 2017 28709880

Bikson M, Paneri B, Mourdoukoutas A, et al: Limited output transcranial electrical stimulation (LOTES-2017): engineering principles, regulatory statutes, and industry standards for wellness, over-the-counter, or prescription devices with low risk. Brain Stimul 11(1):134–157, 2018 29122535

Borckardt JJ, Reeves ST, Milliken C, et al: Prefrontal versus motor cortex transcranial direct current stimulation (tDCS) effects on postsurgical opioid use. Brain Stimul 10(6):1096–1101, 2017 28917592

Brunoni AR, Nitsche MA, Bolognini N, et al: Clinical research with transcranial direct current stimulation (tDCS): challenges and future directions. Brain Stimul 5(3):175–195, 2012 22037126

Castillo-Saavedra L, Gebodh N, Bikson M, et al: Clinically effective treatment of fibromyalgia pain with high-definition transcranial direct current stimulation: phase II open-label dose optimization. J Pain 17(1):14–26, 2016 26456677

Feighner JP, Brown SL, Olivier JE: Electrosleep therapy. A controlled double blind study. J Nerv Ment Dis 157(2):121–128, 1973 4724809

Fregni F, Pascual-Leone A: Technology insight: noninvasive brain stimulation in neurology-perspectives on the therapeutic potential of rTMS and tDCS. Nat Clin Pract Neurol 3(7):383–393, 2007 17611487

Fridriksson J, Elm J, Stark BC, et al: BDNF genotype and tDCS interaction in aphasia treatment. Brain Stimul 11(6):1276–1281, 2018a 30150003

Fridriksson J, Rorden C, Elm J, et al: Transcranial direct current stimulation vs sham stimulation to treat aphasia after stroke: a randomized clinical trial. JAMA Neurol 2018b 30128538 Epub ahead of print

George MS: Reanimating the face: early writings by Duchenne and Darwin on the neurology of facial emotion expression. J Hist Neurosci 3(1):21–33, 1994 11618803

Glaser J, Reeves ST, Stoll WD, et al: Motor/prefrontal transcranial direct current stimulation (tDCS) following lumbar surgery reduces postoperative analgesia use. Spine 41(10):835–839, 2016 26909844

Gomez E, Mikhail AR: Treatment of methadone withdrawal with cerebral electrotherapy (electrosleep). Br J Psychiatry 134:111–113, 1979 760910

Landgrebe M, Hajak G, Wolf S, et al: 1-Hz rTMS in the treatment of tinnitus: a sham-controlled, randomized multicenter trial. Brain Stimul 10(6):1112–1120, 2017 28807845

Liepert J: Motor cortex excitability in stroke before and after constraint-induced movement therapy. Cogn Behav Neurol 19(1):41–47, 2006 16633018

Mulquiney PG, Hoy KE, Daskalakis ZJ, et al: Improving working memory: exploring the effect of transcranial random noise stimulation and transcranial direct current stimulation on the dorsolateral prefrontal cortex. Clin Neurophysiol 122(12):2384–2389, 2011 21665534

Nitsche MA, Doemkes S, Karaköse T, et al: Shaping the effects of transcranial direct current stimulation of the human motor cortex. J Neurophysiol 97(4):3109–3117, 2007 17251360

Poreisz C, Boros K, Antal A, et al: Safety aspects of transcranial direct current stimulation concerning healthy subjects and patients. Brain Res Bull 72(4–6):208–214, 2007 17452283

Rahman A, Reato D, Arlotti M, et al: Cellular effects of acute direct current stimulation: somatic and synaptic terminal effects. J Physiol 591(10):2563–2578, 2013 23478132

Scheldrup M, Greenwood PM, McKendrick R, et al: Transcranial direct current stimulation facilitates cognitive multi-task performance differentially depending on anode location and subtask. Front Hum Neurosci 8:665, 2014 25249958

CHAPTER 9

Other Techniques

Now we have reviewed the major brain stimulation techniques that have U.S. Food and Drug Administration (FDA) approval for clinical uses or Class I evidence of efficacy. However, there are numerous other ways of stimulating the nervous system that we still have not discussed. These other techniques all have in common that they electrically or magnetically stimulate the brain or peripheral nervous system, but there are not enough high-quality and critical studies of these techniques to qualify them for an individual chapter. Although most are not part of mainstream medical treatment, clinicians will want to be aware of these techniques because the more astute patients may ask about them.

Transcutaneous Electrical Nerve Stimulation

Transcutaneous electrical nerve stimulation (TENS) units are some of the most widely used stimulation devices. Developed in the late 1970s, they are largely used for pain relief. Like many of the other stimulation devices, they were discovered serendipitously. Researchers were attempting to directly stimulate the spinal cord for pain relief but needed a surface device to trigger the implanted device. They had to test the tolerability of the actual surface electrode and found that pain patients reported improved pain symptoms just from the surface electrical stimulation alone.

How Is It Done?

TENS devices consist of a small battery-powered device attached to electrodes that are applied to the skin, typically over the low back or neck (Figure 9–1). They require a cream to improve skin conductivity. The stimulation parameters can vary widely but typically are frequency 40–150 hertz (Hz), pulse width 10–1,000 microseconds, and amplitude 10–30 milliamperes. The stimulation is usually constant, applied for 20–30 minutes. In some but not all patients the pain relief is quick and parameter and dose dependent.

What Does It Do to the Brain?

The most widely held theory concerning TENS follows the gate theory of pain and reasons that the skin electrical stimulation preferentially activates low-threshold myelinated nerve fibers, which then inhibit propagation of nociception carried in the smaller unmyelinated C-fibers in the dorsal horn. Studies in animals support this idea.

Is TENS Safe?

TENS is relatively safe unless applied over other nervous tissue, such as the eyes.

Critical Review of Clinical Applications

Interestingly, despite widespread use, the randomized controlled trial data on the use of TENS for low back pain are mixed and rather

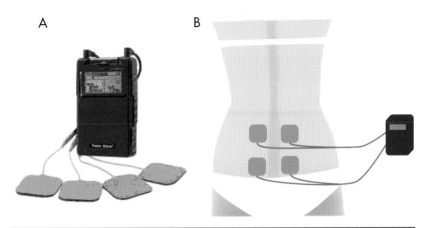

FIGURE 9-1. Transcutaneous electrical nerve stimulation. The battery-powered TENS unit **(A)** generates high-frequency cycling direct current that passes through electrodes placed over the lower back **(B)** or any other peripheral location where the patient has been experiencing pain.

modest. For example, the conservative Cochrane Collaboration, which evaluates treatments, found mixed results for TENS for low-back pain. (Milne et al. 2001). There has been one large study with positive findings, but another large study had negative results.

Electroacupuncture

Electroacupuncture is the application of electrical current to acupuncture needles.

How Is It Done?

Acupuncture is a form of traditional Chinese medicine that seeks to restore health by inserting and manipulating needles in specific points along established ancient meridians. The effectiveness of acupuncture remains controversial in the scientific community, but the emergence of more randomized controlled trials is increasing our understanding of the benefits and limitations of this procedure. A review concluded that the procedure is effective for some, but not all, conditions (Ernst et al. 2007).

Electroacupuncture follows the same principles as traditional acupuncture, but with the application of a mild alternating electrical current flowing between two needles. The electrical pulses are generated by devices that send a small signal to the needles. The current is usually less than 0.6 milliamperes, which is about the same as what is generated by a wristwatch battery. However, the voltage is usually between 40 volts and 80 volts and can spike as high as 130 volts. The duration of a treatment session is usually 10–20 minutes.

What Does It Do to the Nervous System?

Electroacupuncture is intended to provide continuous stimulation, which alleviates the need of the practitioner from constantly manipulating the needles. However, exactly what electroacupuncture does to the nervous system remains unanswered.

Is Electroacupuncture Safe?

Patients are aware of a sensation with electroacupuncture. With the voltage set too high, patients can experience muscle twitching, numbness, and pain. One review of electroacupuncture devices noted that some of the output is erratic and beyond the manufacturer's specifications. The authors concluded that practitioners must be adequately trained to use the electrostimulators safely (Lytle et al. 2000).

Critical Review of Clinical Applications

In general, there are numerous small studies reported in alternative medicine journals describing positive outcomes for electroacupuncture. Pain is the condition most commonly treated. The methodological limitations of these studies make it difficult to determine the utility of the electroacupuncture for Western medicine.

The Cochrane Collaboration evaluated electroacupuncture for control of chemotherapy-induced nausea and vomiting as well as for treatment of rheumatoid arthritis. In both cases the reviewers concluded that there appeared to be some benefit but that the effect was not robust. Likewise, the small size of the limited number of studies precludes recommending electroacupuncture for these conditions (Casimiro et al. 2005; Ezzo et al. 2006).

Cranial Electrotherapy Stimulation

Cranial electrotherapy stimulation (CES) is another form of electrical current applied to the peripheral skin in order to influence the brain. CES is sometimes called "electrosleep," or "cranial electrosleep," because it can make a user sleepy or "spacey" during the stimulation.

One device is commercially marketed in the United States as Alpha-Stim and has received a great deal of publicity recently. The devices are FDA approved for anxiety, insomnia, or depression because they were grandfathered in when the Medical Device Amendments to the FD&C Act were passed in 1976. CES, like electroconvulsive therapy (ECT), which was also grandfathered in, has not been examined the way vagus nerve stimulation, transcranial magnetic stimulation, or the antidepressant medications have. Unlike ECT, CES has not been subjected to any large, multicenter, randomized, blinded studies.

How Is It Done?

One form of CES involves applying a pulsed, low-amplitude electrical current to the head using electrodes clipped to the earlobes (see Figure 9–2). Another involves placing electrodes on the forehead. Still another involves a headband-like device that looks like the visual device Geordi used for seeing on *Star Trek: The Next Generation*. The current comes from a battery source that looks like a TENS device but has a high-frequency cycling design. Thus, using the nomenclature adopted for this book, CES is a specific type of transcutaneous alternating current, because the pulse is bidirectional. The user can increase the intensity from 10 up to 500 millionths of an ampere, but the frequency is set at 0.5 Hz. Because CES generates an alternating bidirectional current, it does not matter which ear is the anode or cathode. The standard session lasts 20 minutes per day but can go as long as 60 minutes if needed.

What Does It Do to the Brain?

Promotional descriptions of CES show the current flowing between the electrodes and traveling through the brain stem, where it stimulates the release of important neurotransmitters. This is more specu-

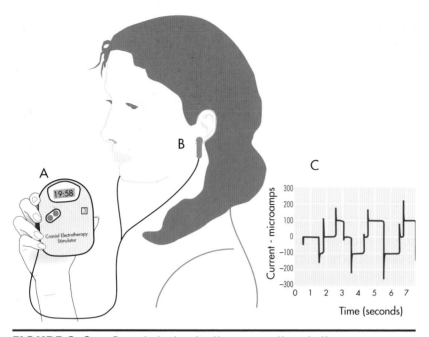

FIGURE 9–2.   Cranial electrotherapy stimulation.

The CES device **(A)** sends the stimulation to the electrodes attached to the patient's ear lobes **(B)**. The stimulation is an alternating current measured in microamperes **(C)**.

lation than actual science. However, in a series of studies, Shealy et al. (1989) found that in patients with treatment-resistant depression, CES was associated with significant elevations in plasma serotonin. Likewise, in nondepressed volunteers, 20 minutes of CES produced significant increases in cerebrospinal fluid serotonin and beta-endorphins and increases in plasma endorphins.

CES treatment also alters electroencephalographic (EEG) readings (Kirsch and Smith 2000). In studies of macaque monkeys, alpha EEG waves were slowed following CES; the slowing was associated with a reduction in adverse reactions to stressful stimuli (Jarzembski 1985). Schroeder and Barr (2001) published a double-blind study on EEG changes in 28 healthy male subjects who underwent sham CES, 0.5-Hz CES, and 100-Hz CES treatment in random order. Both active CES treatments resulted in a downward shift in the alpha mean frequency, with the 100-Hz treatment producing more overall effect and additionally decreasing the beta power fraction.

Is CES Safe?

Many patients will experience mild dizziness, vertigo, and sometimes anxiety or nausea when they start the device. These effects are dose dependent, and generally treatment is applied at a setting that is tolerable. In some CES studies, patients have noted headache, skin irritation (e.g., burns), and lightheadedness or vertigo during or following treatment. Activation is described as a potential side effect in the brochure, but frank mania or hypomania is not mentioned.

Critical Review of Clinical Applications

It is difficult to provide a measured assessment of the clinical studies of the CES device, because there are numerous small studies in nontraditional journals for a maddeningly wide variety of psychiatric and neurological conditions. In general, the devices seem to promote "stress reduction." As such, the best use of the device may be for anxiety, depression, and insomnia. However, there are reports of CES benefiting fibromyalgia, headaches, tremor, attention-deficit/hyperactivity disorder, and cognitive dysfunction as well as substance abuse withdrawal.

Although many studies on CES have been published in the past 40 years, most have used relatively small samples, in which only a dozen or so patients received the active treatment. In addition, the frequency and duration of CES treatment have not been established for different conditions. While short-term CES (e.g., one to five treatments of 23–30 minutes each) may help with acute anxiety, some researchers argue that chronic conditions may require longer periods of treatment (Jarzembski 1985) and that effective therapy for patients with clinical depression or anxiety disorders may only result from daily CES for 2–4 weeks.

The lack of negative studies reported in the literature is troublesome. With the possible exception of exercise or getting a pet, few interventions in medicine are uniformly effective. Either this device is the next aspirin, or some bias is distorting the reports.

To our knowledge, Klawansky et al. (1995) have published the only meta-analysis of CES—and that was more than two decades ago. They reviewed randomized controlled trials of CES for anxiety, brain dysfunction, headache, and insomnia. A total of eight trials on anxiety were combined, and effect sizes were used to compare outcome measures. Overall, CES was significantly more effective than sham treatment (effect size, 0.62), although placebo effects may have been a factor because many patients who received sham therapy also improved (30%) (Klawansky et al. 1995).

Summary of Clinical Use

A simple "stress reducing" device that patients can use at home would be a welcome addition to modern medicine. CES looks appealing with numerous positive studies for a wide range of disorders. The technique is relatively inexpensive, easy to operate, and apparently safe. However, the studies are small and of poor quality. It is hard to know whether the treatment is truly effective or a modern snake oil. Rigorous academic studies are needed.

Stimulating Spiritual Growth?

Sometimes it is hard to separate the wheat from the chaff in this dynamic field of brain stimulation. However, we think this next device goes too far. Dr. Persinger has developed a device (the 8-coil Shakti) that generates a weak magnetic field over the temporal lobes (see Figure 9–3). The magnets alternate between the green and blue, which generates a changing magnetic current over the brain. Remarkably, this device is supposed to induce spiritual growth and well-being. We will await the results of the randomized controlled trial before purchasing ours.

Other Techniques

We close this chapter with a quick review of some techniques about which the informed clinician should be aware.

Sacral nerve stimulation (SNS; also known as InterStim therapy) is a technique used to control fecal or urinary incontinence. The stimulating electrodes are placed in the spinal cord (S3 fora-

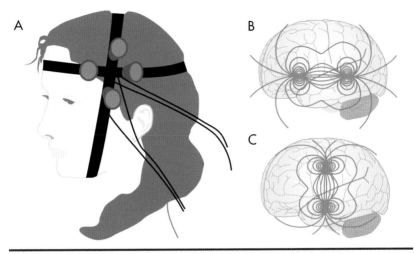

FIGURE 9–3. Shakti device.

The 8-coil Shakti consists of four magnets strapped to each side of the head **(A)**. The magnetic signal alternates between the *green* and the *blue*, which generates different magnetic fields over the brain (**B** and **C**). This device is believed to enhance religious experiences.

men) near the sacral nerve, and the generator is placed subcutaneously in the buttock. Generally, physicians perform a challenge or screening stimulation before implanting the full device into the nerve. It is not known exactly how SNS improves overall control of incontinence, other than by resetting tone and spinal cord control over voiding or defecation.

Recent research suggests, but has not proven, that *percutaneous tibial nerve stimulation*, or PTNS, might also be effective in treating incontinence. A recent open-label study from the Netherlands and Italy found in 35 patients that 12 weeks of once-weekly treatment reduced incontinence. The stimulation was applied using needle electrodes to the posterior tibial nerve in the shank at 20 Hz for 30 minutes per session. Sixty-three percent of the patients found this helpful and chose to continue the treatment after the formal trial ended. The recent work builds on prior work done by a now defunct company called UroSurge.

Another class of interventions that fit under some definition of brain stimulation comprise devices that employ very-low-level electrical stimulation. These are basically TENS devices operating at very low amplitude. These forms of stimulation are known as *microcurrent electrical neuromuscular stimulation*, or MENS, and *transcutaneous low-voltage microamperage stimulation*, or tLVMAS. There are really no good studies regarding the efficacy of these devices in any conditions. They are likely generally safe, however. They are used occasionally as well to promote bone regeneration or other forms of healing.

References

Casimiro L, Barnsley L, Brosseau L, et al: Acupuncture and electroacupuncture for the treatment of rheumatoid arthritis. Cochrane Database Syst Rev (4):CD003788, 2005 16235342

Ernst E, Pittler MH, Wider B, et al: Acupuncture: its evidence-base is changing. Am J Chin Med 35(1):21–25, 2007 17265547

Ezzo JM, Richardson MA, Vickers A, et al: Acupuncture-point stimulation for chemotherapy-induced nausea or vomiting. Cochrane Database Syst Rev (2):CD002285, 2006 16625560

Jarzembski WB: Electrical stimulation and substance abuse treatment. Neurobehav Toxicol Teratol 7(2):119–123, 1985 3889683

Kirsch DL, Smith RB: The use of cranial electrotherapy stimulation in the management of chronic pain: a review. NeuroRehabilitation 14(2):85–94, 2000 11455071

Klawansky S, Yeung A, Berkey C, et al: Meta-analysis of randomized controlled trials of cranial electrostimulation. Efficacy in treating selected psychological and physiological conditions. J Nerv Ment Dis 183(7):478–484, 1995 7623022

Lytle CD, Thomas BM, Gordon EA, et al: Electrostimulators for acupuncture: safety issues. J Altern Complement Med 6(1):37–44, 2000 10706234

Milne S, Welch V, Brosseau L, et al: Transcutaneous electrical nerve stimulation (TENS) for chronic low back pain. Cochrane Database Syst Rev (2):CD003008, 2001 11406059

Schroeder MJ, Barr RE: Quantitative analysis of the electroencephalogram during cranial electrotherapy stimulation. Clin Neurophysiol 112(11):2075–2083, 2001 11682346

Shealy CN, Cady R, Wilkie RG, et al: Depression: a diagnostic, neurochemical profile and therapy with cranial electrotherapy stimulation (CES). J Neurol Orthop Med Surg 10(4):319–321, 1989

CHAPTER 10

Future Techniques

In this closing chapter we are going to predict the future. In the future everyone will travel in flying cars. (More likely, we will struggle with intolerable heat, devastating storms, and a biomass clogged with plastic.) However, if we are able to forestall ecological disaster, we believe the future is bright for brain stimulation therapies.

Since Cerletti's first use of electroconvulsive therapy (ECT) in 1938, several themes have emerged in the field of brain stimulation. These include gradual decreases in stimulation intensity, greater focality of treatment, increased specificity of brain stimulation targets, and wider public acceptance of therapeutic neuromodulation—in addition to the development of new technologies. A hallmark feature of neuromodulation over the past 80 years is the declining invasiveness of stimulation, combined with focal anatomic precision. In this vein, we close out this book by discussing two emerging less-invasive methods: low-intensity focused ultrasound pulsation (LIFUP) and temporally interfering electric fields. These each have the potential to noninvasively stimulate focal locations deep in the brain—without surgery or leaving hardware in the brain.

Low-Intensity Focused Ultrasound Pulsation

LIFUP uses sound to stimulate the brain. To do this, you place either a single large, concave-shaped or multiple ultrasound transducers on the scalp. These "speakers" produce high-frequency (100-hertz [Hz]) sound pulses (*sonications*), typically for 30 seconds at a time for 10 trains of pulses. Unlike traditional ultrasound, which constantly transmits ultrasound and "listens" to the echo to form an image, LIFUP delivers the ultrasound in packets, or pulses. Bones typically block ultrasound waves, but for reasons that are not clear, pulsed ultrasound causes neurons to depolarize and fire (see Figure 10–1). Apparently, it is possible to deliver the ultrasound from multiple sources and use the skull as a lens to shape and focus the convergent beam deeper in the brain. The clinical and research use of LIFUP thus incorporates structural magnetic resonance imaging (MRI) scans taken before stimulation in order to position and calculate how multiple ultrasonic pulsations will converge at a location in the brain (taking into account the bone dispersion of the beam from the skull). Because each transducer cannot individually cause neuronal discharge, neuronal firing can be focused both deep (2–12 centimeters [cm] under the cap; for comparison, traditional transcranial magnetic stimulation [TMS] can stimulate 1–3.4 cm^2 deep; Deng et al. 2013; Hanlon 2017) and focally (as small as 0.5 millimeters [mm] in diameter), and up to 1,000 mm; the focality of a standard, commercially available 70-mm figure-eight coil is roughly 50 mm^2 (Deng et al. 2013; Hanlon 2017). Interestingly, the pulse width of the carrying frequency of LIFUP (0.5 milliseconds) is strikingly similar to that

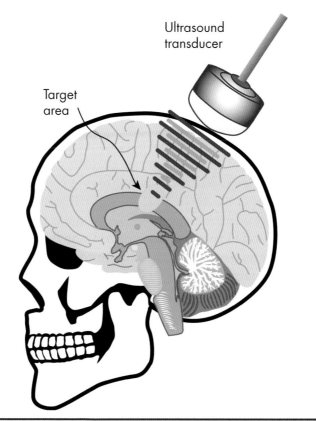

Ultrasound transducer

Target area

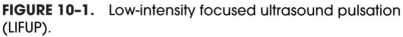

FIGURE 10–1. Low-intensity focused ultrasound pulsation (LIFUP).

LIFUP uses the skull to focus ultrasound pulsations deep in the brain.

used in all other pulsed neuromodulation therapies (deep brain stimulation [DBS] 0.6 milliseconds; ECT: 0.5 milliseconds; TMS: 0.2 milliseconds; vagus nerve stimulation [VNS]: 0.5 milliseconds), suggesting that this timeframe is mechanistically meaningful. This is a good example of the common background science of brain stimulation that transcends the individual methods.

It is important to differentiate LIFUP from ultrasound ablation. Neurosurgeons use much higher amounts of ultrasound focused in a beam in order to actually produce lesions. Lesioning the thalamus with ultrasound ablation is now approved by the U.S. Food and Drug Administration (FDA).

Researchers have examined the effects of LIFUP in preclinical and clinical settings. Studies are confirming the ability of LIFUP, affectionately called *sonication,* to safely stimulate neural tissue (Min et al. 2011; Tufail et al. 2010; Tyler et al. 2008; Yoo et al. 2011), and cellular mechanisms for its efficacy have been proposed (Choi et al. 2013; Krasovitski et al. 2011; Min et al. 2011; Plaksin et al. 2014; Tyler et al. 2008; Wahab et al. 2012; Yang et al. 2012). Recent studies are exploring benefits of LIFUP in human patients (Schiff et al. 2007). Monti et al. (2016) described a case study in which they used LIFUP to stimulate a comatose patient's thalamus (Schiff et al. 2007). Two pre-LIFUP assessments rated the patient as being in a minimally conscious state. After sonication, the patient recovered some motor functions the following day, including full language comprehension and communication by nodding and shaking his head. Five days post-LIFUP, the patient attempted to walk. Although this study was neither blinded nor sham controlled, the first application of therapeutic LIFUP in a human patient was encouraging. We expect more therapeutic applications of LIFUP and potential clinical trials in the future. If sonication continues to show clinical potential, it has the potential to supplant the role of DBS without the need for surgery! However, DBS offers the advantage of continuous stimulation—24/7. Obviously, patients cannot wear a LIFUP helmet home. Alternatively, if we can learn to stimulate in a manner that results in enduring changes to the behavioral circuits, we may be able to substitute several sessions of LIFUP, rewire the brain, and throw away the hardware. LIFUP can certainly stimulate deep and focused without neurosurgery and thus may be a key next step in the field of brain stimulation.

Temporally Interfering Electric Fields

Grossman et al. (2017) at MIT recently pioneered an alternative brain stimulation approach that can noninvasively stimulate deep in the brain (at least in mice). This method, called *temporally interfering electric fields* (or *temporal interference* [TI]), utilizes very-high-frequency (≥1,000-Hz) oscillating electric fields applied at multiple locations on the scalp. TI has the capacity to stimulate neurons *only* at the point the electrical fields converge deep in the brain. Very-high-frequency stimulation will not directly cause neuronal firing because all neurons (even in nonprimates) appear to apply a low-pass filter to electrical signals from the neural membrane (i.e., very-high-frequency stimulation *does not* stimulate) (Hutcheon and Yarom 2000). Creatively drawing on this principle, Grossman's team applied two temporally interfering electrical fields to each side of a transgenic mouse's head, with each electrical field differing by only 10 Hz (sinusoidal currents at 2,010 Hz and 2,000 Hz). They found that at the point where the electric fields intersected, the effective stimulation frequency was the difference between the two higher frequencies (10 Hz)—which *can* stimulate the neurons. Thus, they effectively applied 10-Hz stimulation deep in the brain, where the two different waves met and interacted. Figures 10–2A and 10–2B schematically show how high frequency waves can combine to form waves of higher amplitude and lower frequency.

The MIT group demonstrated that this method could noninvasively stimulate deep brain regions in the mouse like the hippocampus. Like LIFUP, TI has the potential to treat brain disorders for which stimulation of a deep pathological locus might matter. Although no studies to date have investigated the use of TI in humans or animal disease models, barring some unexpected safety issue, TI may have translational applications in the near future. (Some researchers, however, are questioning whether this approach will actually work in a much larger human brain, with the increased volume of tissue. The intensity of current applied may need to be very high, perhaps similar to ECT. If this is true, one would likely have to perform TI under anesthesia, limiting to some degree the clinical and research applications. Figure 10–2C shows how this might look in the human brain.)

A Word About Biomarkers

Much to our great frustration, we continue to be unable to "see" mental illness. Despite all the expensive scanners that can look

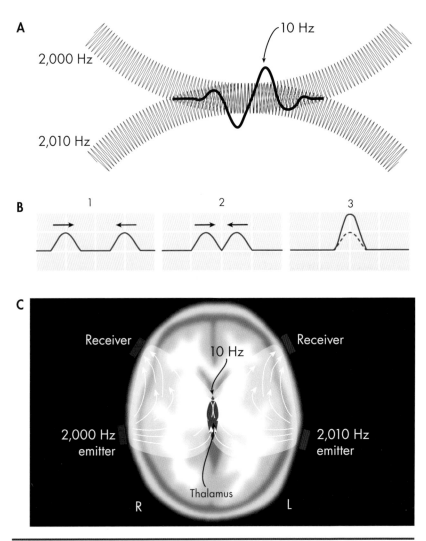

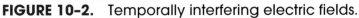

FIGURE 10–2. Temporally interfering electric fields.

(A) When two electrical fields with slightly different frequencies merge, a low-frequency electrical impulse is generated. (B) When two electrical impulses meet, the amplitude is the combination of the two. (C) Two high-frequency electrical fields only stimulate the neurons where they meet and overlap—at the thalamus.

deep into the brain, we still do not have a lab test or imaging study that can diagnose mental illness. Positron emission tomography scans, single-photon emission tomography scans, functional magnetic resonance imaging—nothing!

The current interest is networks. The neuroscience community believes that emotions, cognition, and behavior are conceived and initiated by networks of neurons communicating across the brain. Depression, anxiety, attention-deficit/hyperactivity disorder, eating disorders, and so on are the product not of a faulty cluster of neurons but of some dysfunction in a network. Okay, that makes sense, but how do we visualize or measure these networks?

With networks the state of the art is *functional connectivity:* an indirect measure of brain networks. Functional connectivity analyzes correlation in activity. So, if the motor cortex and the visual cortex are repeatedly active at the same time (which is measured by a functional MRI and some serious number crunching), then these two regions are assumed to be part of a network. Typically, the functional connectivity analysis is done while the subject is quietly resting. The most famous network is the *default mode network,* which is active when subjects are awake but resting and day dreaming…with their head in a scanner. This has led to one of the premier questions in mental health and neuroscience: Can analysis of functional connectivity be used to determine mental health treatments?

Fox et al. (2012) were some of the first to test how the TMS target for clinically treated depression patients using the 5-cm rule, and its functional connectivity to the subgenual cingulate, differed between responders and nonresponders. Their research group found that the more effective stimulation site was significantly more anticorrelated with the subgenual cingulate, suggesting that these results could be prospectively applied to determine the best possible stimulation target. Prospective applications of these findings have confirmed that higher anticorrelation between the dorsolateral prefrontal cortex and subgenual cingulate correlates with better response to TMS for depression and that TMS changes the connectivity between the default mode network and the frontoparietal central execution network (Liston et al. 2014).

In the future, we expect more research in the area of how neuroimaging can prospectively influence stimulation targets as the field of neuromodulation trends toward more refinement and higher individualization of treatment. It will be interesting to see if neuropsychiatrists someday base stimulation targets on each individual's intrinsic functional connectivity. Although this is theoretically feasible, an MRI scan for each patient may be prohibitively expensive for most indications.

Building on what Fox and others have found, Drysdale et al. (2017) set out to identify different biotypes (i.e., neurophysiological subtypes based on different patterns of dysfunctional connectivity in limbic and frontostriatal networks) in depression. To do this, the authors applied a machine learning algorithm that clustered patients into distinct groups based on whole-brain patterns of abnormal functional connectivity. This identified two groups of network patterns that involved either frontal/orbitofrontal areas or the limbic system (amygdala, subgenual cingulate, lateral prefrontal cortex, ventral hippocampus, and ventral striatum). On top of core depressive symptoms, the researchers identified which connectivity features correlated with different items on the Hamilton Depression Rating Scale (Ham-D) and further delineated the depressive subtypes into four biotypes.

On top of core clinical features of depression that the four biotypes shared (e.g., low mood, anhedonia, fatigue, and lack of energy that are associated with the insula, orbitofrontal cortex, ventromedial prefrontal cortex, and various subcortical areas), the biotypes differed on other clinical symptoms. Notably, types 1 and 4 had increased anxiety, types 3 and 4 had greater anhedonia and psychomotor slowing, and types 1 and 2 had lower energy and more fatigue—all of which were significantly correlated with brain activity in affiliated regions. Most intriguing to the field of neuromodulation, the authors identified which biotypes responded best to 10-Hz clinical repetitive TMS, which greatly differed among groups. While the majority of biotype 1 (82.5%) and biotype 3 (61.0%) patients had a 25% or greater reduction in their Ham-D scores from TMS, only 25.0% and 29.6% in biotypes 2 and 4 showed similar improvements. Moving forward, we expect that the push toward greater individualization of treatment will continue. If it is not currently feasible to have each patient get an MRI scan prior to treatment, perhaps biotyping based on Ham-D responses could assist in identifying which patients will respond to which location or type of treatment. Notably, clinical symptoms did not track well with the imaging-defined biotypes.

Summary

The field of brain stimulation is growing rapidly, with new methods emerging each year and new FDA-approved treatments happening almost monthly. It is likely that in 10 years there will be new brain stimulation treatments not even conceived of at this moment. These brain stimulation methods are comfortably becoming the third arm of psychiatric treatment, settling in beside talking therapies and medications.

References

Choi JB, Lim SH, Cho KW, et al: The Effect of Focused Ultrasonic Stimulation on the Activity of Hippocampal Neurons in Multi-Channel Electrode. Paper presented at Neural Engineering (NER) 6th International IEEE/EMBS Conference, San Diego, CA, November 6–8, 2013

Deng ZD, Lisanby SH, Peterchev AV: Electric field depth-focality tradeoff in transcranial magnetic stimulation: simulation comparison of 50 coil designs. Brain Stimul 6(1):1–13, 2013 22483681

Drysdale AT, Grosenick L, Downar J, et al: Resting-state connectivity biomarkers define neurophysiological subtypes of depression. Nat Med 23(1):28–38, 2017 27918562

Fox MD, Buckner RL, White MP, et al: Efficacy of transcranial magnetic stimulation targets for depression is related to intrinsic functional connectivity with the subgenual cingulate. Biol Psychiatry 72(7):595–603, 2012 22658708

Grossman N, Bono D, Dedic N, et al: Noninvasive deep brain stimulation via temporally interfering electric fields. Cell 169(6):1029–1041, 2017 28575667

Hanlon C: Blunt or precise? A note about the relative precision of figure-of-eight rTMS coils. Brain Stimul 10(2):338–339, 2017 28126249

Hutcheon B, Yarom Y: Resonance, oscillation and the intrinsic frequency preferences of neurons. Trends Neurosci 23(5):216–222, 2000 10782127

Krasovitski B, Frenkel V, Shoham S, et al: Intramembrane cavitation as a unifying mechanism for ultrasound-induced bioeffects. Proc Natl Acad Sci USA 108(8):3258–3263, 2011 21300891

Liston C, Chen AC, Zebley BD, et al: Default mode network mechanisms of transcranial magnetic stimulation in depression. Biol Psychiatry 76(7):517–526, 2014 24629537

Min BK, Yang PS, Bohlke M, et al: Focused ultrasound modulates the level of cortical neurotransmitters: potential as a new functional brain mapping technique. Int J Imaging Syst Technol 21(2):232–240, 2011

Monti MM, Schnakers C, Korb AS: Non-invasive ultrasonic thalamic stimulation in disorders of consciousness after severe brain injury: a first-in-man report. Brain Stimul 9(6):940–941, 2016 27567470

Plaksin M, Shoham S, Kimmel E: Intramembrane cavitation as a predictive bio-piezoelectric mechanism for ultrasonic brain stimulation. Phys Rev X 4(1):011004, 2014

Schiff ND, Giacino JT, Kalmar K, et al: Behavioural improvements with thalamic stimulation after severe traumatic brain injury. Nature 448(7153):600–603, 2007 17671503

Tufail Y, Matyushov A, Baldwin N, et al: Transcranial pulsed ultrasound stimulates intact brain circuits. Neuron 66(5):681–694, 2010 20547127

Tyler WJ, Tufail Y, Finsterwald M, et al: Remote excitation of neuronal circuits using low-intensity, low-frequency ultrasound. PLoS One 3(10):e3511, 2008 18958151

Wahab RA, Choi M, Liu Y, et al: Mechanical bioeffects of pulsed high intensity focused ultrasound on a simple neural model. Med Phys 39(7 part 1):4274–4283, 2012 22830761

Yang PS, Kim H, Lee W, et al: Transcranial focused ultrasound to the thalamus is associated with reduced extracellular GABA levels in rats. Neuropsychobiology 65(3):153–160, 2012 22378299

Yoo S-S, Bystritsky A, Lee J-H, et al: Focused ultrasound modulates region-specific brain activity. Neuroimage 56(3):1267–1275, 2011 21354315

Appendix by Disease

Disease	Class 1 evidence of therapeutic benefit	Some data, but not convincing evidence
Anxiety	TMS (OCD)	CES, TMS, VNS, electroacupuncture
Catatonia		ECT
Depression	ECT, TMS	DBS, VNS, CES, MST, tDCS
Dystonia		DBS
Epilepsy	VNS, RNS	DBS, TMS, ECT
Headache	Cervical VNS (cluster headache) Single-pulse TMS (migraine with aura)	TMS
Incontinence	SNS, PTNS	
Mania	ECT	
Muscle rehabilitation		MENS, tLVMAS
Obesity	VNS (gastric)	
Pain, acute	TMS	tDCS
Pain, chronic		CBS, electroacupuncture, TMS, tDCS
Parkinson's disease	DBS	ECT, TMS, tDCS
Poststroke aphasia	tDCS	
Schizophrenia		TMS, ECT

Appendix by Stimulation Method

Acronym/ Name	Full name	Page
Intentionally produces a seizure		
ECT	Electroconvulsive therapy	45
Electroshock	*See* ECT	
FEAST	Focal electrical alternating current seizure therapy	55
MST	Magnetic seizure therapy	55
Shock therapy	*See* ECT	
Non–seizure producing, but requires surgery for implantation of an electrode		
CBS	Cortical brain stimulation	127
DBS	Deep brain stimulation	121
PTNS	Percutaneous tibial nerve stimulation	167
RNS	Responsive neural stimulation	126
RST	Responsive stimulation therapy	122
SNS	Sacral nerve stimulation	166
VNS	Vagus nerve stimulation	71
Non–seizure producing, surface application of electrode or electromagnet		
CES	Cranial electrotherapy stimulation	163
FEAT	Focal electrical alternating current therapy	153
MENS	Microcurrent electrical neuromuscular stimulation	168
tACS	Transcranial alternating current stimulation	152
tDCS	Transcranial direct current stimulation	147
TENS	Transcutaneous electrical nerve stimulation	160
tLVMAS	Transcutaneous low-voltage microamperage stimulation	168
TMS	Transcranial magnetic stimulation	95
rTMS	Repetitive transcranial magnetic stimulation	100

Index

Page numbers printed in **boldface** type refer to tables or figures.

Action potential, 33

Acupuncture, 161

Addictions, and transcranial magnetic stimulation, 116

Adverse events. *See* Side effects

Afferent fibers, of vagus nerve, **83**

Age, and electroconvulsive therapy, 49, 61

Aggression, brain stimulation and inhibition of, 10. *See also* Behavior

ALICNA (anterior lining of the internal capsule, nucleus accumbens), and deep brain stimulation, 141–142

Alpha-Stim, 163

Alphatron 4000, **22**

Alternating current, 18–20, **21, 22**. *See also* Transcranial alternating current stimulation

Alternative medicine acupuncture and, 161
vagus stimulation and, **84**

American Psychiatric Association, 47, 60, 63–64

Amperes, 15

Anesthesia
deep brain stimulation and, 124
electroconvulsive therapy and, 56–57

Anhedonia, and emotional pacemaker, 8

Animal magnetism, **98**

Anodal transcranial direct current stimulation, 148, 150–151

Anterior cingulate cortex, and transcranial magnetic stimulation, 108

Anticonvulsant effect, of electroconvulsive therapy on brain, 58–59

Antidepressants, efficacy of compared with electroconvulsive therapy, 64, 65

Anti-inflammatory effects, of vagus nerve stimulation, 92

Antipsychotics
electroconvulsive therapy and introduction of, 47, 65–66
reduction in need for neurosurgery and, 122

Anxiety
cranial electrotherapy stimulation and, 165, 166
vagus nerve stimulation and, 91

Aphasia. *See also* Speech therapy
transcranial magnetic stimulation and, 117
vagus nerve stimulation and, 80, 91

AspireSR, 78

Asystole, and vagus nerve stimulation surgery, 85–86

Atom, structure of, 14, **15**

Attention-deficit/hyperactivity disorder (ADHD), **43**

Auditory hallucinations, and transcranial magnetic stimulation for schizophrenia, 113

Auricular branch of the vagus nerve (ABVN), 79

Autobiographical memory, and electroconvulsive therapy, 61

Axon hillock, 33, 34, 36–37, **38**

Bailey, P., 72

Barbiturates, 57

Barker, Anthony, 99

Basal ganglia, and Parkinson's disease, 129, **131**

Battery, 14–15, **16**

Behavior. *See also* Aggression; Impulsive behavior

  pairing of vagus nerve stimulation with, 79

  transcranial magnetic stimulation and research on mechanisms of, 117–118

Benabid, A. L., 122–123

Berger, Hans, 39

Beta waves, and deep brain stimulation for Parkinson's disease, **131**

Bilateral placement, of electrodes, 50–52

Biomarkers, for mental illness, 173, 175–177

Bipolar delivery, of electrical pulse, 27–28

Bipolar depression, and electro-convulsive therapy, 64, 65

Bipolar disorder, and vagus nerve stimulation, 87

Boston Scientific, 140

Bottom-up stimulation, and vagus nerve stimulation, 82

Brain

  background electrical activity in, 28

  conductivity of tissues, 17

  cranial electrotherapy stimulation and, 163–164

  deep brain stimulation and, 128–31, 132, **137**

  electroconvulsive therapy and, 54, 58–60

  electrical and chemical communication in, 1, **2**

  electroencephalography and, 38–42, **43**

  generation of action potential, 34–38

  intracellular charge, 31–32

  transcranial direct current stimulation and, 149–152

  transcranial magnetic stimulation and, 106–108

  vagus nerve stimulation and, **75**, 82–85

  transcutaneous electrical nerve stimulation and, 160

Brain chips, and history of brain stimulation, 10–11

Brain-derived neurotrophic factor (BDNF), 59

Brain stimulation. *See also* Clinical applications; Deep brain stimulation; Electroconvulsive therapy; Low-intensity focused ultrasound pulsation; Transcranial direct current stimulation; Transcranial magnetic stimulation; Vagus nerve stimulation
current research on, xiii–xi
determination of correct dose, 28–30
discoveries in neuroscience in twentieth century, ix–xi
electricity and parameters for, 22–28
electrochemical communication in brain and new treatment options, 2–3
emergence of themes in field of, 169–170
history of, 3–11
resistance in, 17
side effects of as different from conventional treatments, xiv
Brainsway company, **104, 105,** 112, 113
Bremer, F., 72
Brief pulse waveform, 52

Cardiac arrest, and vagus nerve stimulation, 80
Cardiac arrhythmias, 62
Cardiac pacemakers, 122
Cardiovascular side effects, of electroconvulsive therapy, 62
Cardioverter-defibrillator, 122
Catatonia, and electroconvulsive therapy, 64, 65

Cathodal transcranial direct current stimulation, 148, 150, 151
Cells, structure of nerve, 33, **35**
Cerlitti, Ugo, 45–47
Cervical vagus nerve stimulation, 76–77
CES. *See* Cranial electrotherapy stimulation
Charcot, Jean-Martin, 147
Charge density, 29
Chemical imbalance, use of term, 1–2
Chemical signal, and action potential, 37–38
Chemotherapy, and electroacupuncture, 162
China, and traditional medicine, 161
Chlorpromazine, 47
Chronaxie, **49**
Chronic heart failure, and vagus nerve stimulation, 80
Clinical applications, of brain stimulation
cranial electrotherapy stimulation and, 165–166
deep brain stimulation and, 132–144
electroacupuncture and, 162
electroconvulsive therapy and, 63–68
transcranial direct current stimulation and, 153–157
transcutaneous electrical nerve stimulation and, 160–161
transcranial magnetic stimulation and, 110–118
vagus nerve stimulation and, 87–92

Closed loop feedback, and vagus
    nerve stimulation, 78, 88
Closed-loop smart deep brain
    stimulation devices, **131**
Closed loop stimulation, and
    EEG data, 42
Clozapine, 66
Cluster headaches, and vagus
    nerve stimulation, 90–91
Cochrane Collaboration, 161, 162
Cognition, and cognitive
    impairment. *See also* Memory
    deep brain stimulation and,
        131–132
    electroconvulsive therapy
        and, 60–62
    transcranial magnetic
        stimulation and, **109**
    vagus nerve stimulation and,
        87
Conductivity, and resistance, 17
Congestive heart failure, and
    vagus nerve stimulation, **87**
Constant high-frequency deep
    brain stimulation, 128
Constant theta burst (cTBS), 105
Constraint induced movement
    therapy, 154
Continuation treatment, with
    electroconvulsive therapy,
    66–68
Cortical brain stimulation, 127–128
Cortical silent period, and
    transcranial magnetic
    stimulation, 117
Cranial electrotherapy
    stimulation (CES), 163–166
cTBS. *See* Constant theta burst
Current, and principles of
    electricity, 15, 16, 17
Current density, 16, 28

Cyberonics Inc., 74
Cycle, of alternating current, 20

DBS. *See* Deep brain stimulation
Deep brain stimulation (DBS)
    clinical applications of,
        132–144
    development of new methods
        of brain stimulation and,
        xi
    effects of on brain, 128–131,
        137
    history of, 121–123
    methodology of, 123–126
    Parkinson's disease and, xiii,
        124–125, 128–131, 132–135
    safety and adverse effects of,
        131–132, 135
Default mode network, 175
Delgado, Jose, 10–11
Delirium, and side effects of
    electroconvulsive therapy,
    61
Dendrites, 33, 34
Depression
    deep brain stimulation for,
        139–142
    electroconvulsive therapy for,
        48, 51, 58, 59, 64–65, 67
    identification of biotypes, 176
    transcranial direct current
        stimulation for, 156
    transcranial magnetic
        stimulation for, 100–101,
        102, 108, 110–113,
        175–176
    vagus nerve stimulation for,
        74, 85, 88–90, 103
Developing countries, and
    electroconvulsive therapy,
    57, 63

Direct current, and principles of electricity, 14–17. *See also* Transcranial direct current stimulation

Directionality, of electrical stimulation, 23

Dizziness, and transcranial direct current stimulation, 152

Dose, and dosing
determination of for brain stimulation, 28–30
electroconvulsive therapy and, 48–50
vagus nerve stimulation and, 80–81

Dose titration, and electroconvulsive therapy, 50

Dry cell, 14. *See also* Battery

DuBois, F., 72

Duchenne de Boulogne, Georges, 147–148, **149**

Duration, of electrical pulse, 25–26

Dystonia, and deep brain stimulation, 123, 124, 136–138

ECT. *See* Electroconvulsive therapy

Edison, Thomas, **20**

EEG. *See* Electroencephalography

Elderly, and side effects of electroconvulsive therapy, 61

Electrical rhythms, and effects of vagus nerve stimulation on brain, 82–83

Electricity
alternating current and, 18–20, **21**, 22
determination of dose for brain stimulation, 28–30

electroencephalography and, 38–42
generation of action potential in brain, 34–38
intracellular charge, 31–32
magnetism and, 18
parameters for brain stimulation, 22–28
review of basic principles, 14–18

Electroacupuncture, 161–162

Electrochemical communication, in brain, 1, **2**

Electroconvulsive therapy (ECT)
anesthesia and, 56–57
clinical applications of, 63–68
for depression, 48, 51, 58, 59
dose and dosing, 29–30, 48–50
effect of on brain, 58–60, 108
electrode placement, 50–52
focal seizures and, 54–56
history of, x, xi, 45–48
location of, 53–54
outdated equipment and nonstandard treatment protocols, **63**
pulse width and, 24–25
question of seizure as necessary for, 58
relevance of resistance in, 17
safety and adverse events of, 60–63, 131
for schizophrenia in developing countries, **57**
transcranial direct current stimulation compared with, **151**
waveforms and, 52–53, **153**

ElectroCore, 78–79

Electrodes
deep brain stimulation and
adjustment or placement
of, 124–125, **126, 135**
electroconvulsive therapy and
placement of, 50–52
Electroencephalography (EEG)
cranial electrotherapy
stimulation and readings
from, 164
electrical activity in brain and,
39–42
history of, 38–39
sleep and, 42–43
Electromagnets, and
electromagnetism, 18, 96–98
Electromotive force, 14. *See also*
Voltage
Electrons, 14, **15**
Electrosleep therapy, 148, 163
Electrostatic pressure, and
intracellular charge, 32, **33**
Emergency shutoff, of cervical
vagus nerve stimulation, 82
Emotional pacemaker, and history
of brain stimulation, 8–9
Epilepsy
deep brain stimulation and, 139
electroconvulsive therapy
and, 66
history of brain stimulation
and, 5–7
vagus nerve stimulation and,
74, **75,** 78, 80, **81,** 85, 88
Essential tremor, and deep brain
stimulation, 135–136
Excitatory neurons, 35, **36, 38**
Exposure therapy, for posttraumatic stress disorder, 116
Extrasensory perception (ESP),
39

Faraday, Michael, 96, 106
Faraday's law, **97**
Fatigue, after transcranial direct
current stimulation, 152
FEAST. *See* Focal electrically
applied seizure therapy
FEAT. *See* Focal electrically
applied therapy
Fish, and history of brain
stimulation, 3, **4**
Flurothyl gas, and seizures, 46
fMRI. *See* Functional magnetic
resonance imaging
Focal electrically applied seizure
therapy (FEAST), 55, **56,** 152,
153
Focal electrically applied therapy
(FEAT), **153**
Focal seizures, and
electroconvulsive therapy,
54–56
Foley, J.O., 72
Food and Drug Administration
(FDA)
approval process for brain
stimulation therapies,
87–88
cranial electrotherapy
stimulation and, 163
deep brain stimulation and,
123, 141
low-intensity focused ultrasound pulsation and, 171
transcranial direct current
stimulation and, 148
transcranial magnetic
stimulation devices and,
101
vagus nerve stimulation
devices and, 74, 78–79,
89–90

Franklin, Benjamin, **98**
Freeman, W., **143**
Frequency, of electrical pulse
    effects of deep brain stimula-
        tion on brain and, 125, 128
    electrical parameters for brain
        stimulation and, 23–24,
        104–106
Freud, Sigmund, ix
Fritsch, Gustav, 5
Frontal lobes, and location of
    electroconvulsive therapy
    seizures, 54
Frontal lobotomies, 121–122, **143**
Functional connectivity, and
    brain networks, 175
Functional magnetic resonance
    imaging (fMRI)
    studies of vagus nerve
        stimulation and, 81
    synchronous neuronal firing
        and, 42

Galen, 3
Galvani, Aldini, **4**
Galvani, Luigi, 3–4
Gamma-aminobutyric acid
    (GABA), and vagus nerve
    stimulation, 84
GammaCore, 78–79, 90–91
Gastric vagus nerve stimulation,
    for obesity, 79, 82, 90
Gender, and electroconvulsive
    therapy, 49
Generators, electric, 19, **21,** 22
George, M. S., 100, 110
Glial cells, and myelin, 37
Globus pallidus interna, and
    deep brain stimulation for
    Parkinson's disease, 130–131,
    133, 137

Glucose metabolism, and
    electroconvulsive therapy, **59**
Goddard, Graham, x
Greece, history of brain
    stimulation in ancient, 3, **4**

Hamilton Depression Rating
    Scale, 51, 100, **101,** 111, 176
Headache. *See also* Migraine
    headaches
    side effects of electroconvul-
        sive therapy and, 63
    side effects of transcranial
        magnetic stimulation and,
        109
    transcranial magnetic
        stimulation for treatment
        of, 115
    vagus nerve stimulation for
        treatment of, 90–91
Hearing loss, as side effect of
    transcranial magnetic
    stimulation, 109
Heart rate, and side effects of
    vagus nerve stimulation,
    86–87. *See also* Cardiac
    arrhythmias; Chronic heart
    failure
Heath, Robert, x, 8–9, 142
Hertz (Hz), 24
Hitzig, Eduard, 5
Hoarseness, as side effect of
    vagus nerve stimulation,
    86
Home use, of transcranial direct
    current stimulation, 156
Hormones, ECT-induced
    seizures and balance of in
    brain, 60
Hypomania, and vagus nerve
    stimulation, 87

Imipramine, 47

Implantable vagus nerve
    stimulation, **81**

Impulse generator, and deep
    brain stimulation, 123, **124**

Impulsive behavior, and deep
    brain stimulation for
    Parkinson's disease, **132**

Incontinence, and percutaneous
    tibial nerve stimulation, 167

Infection, deep brain stimulation
    and risk of, 131

Inhibitory neurons, 35, 36, 38

Insurance companies, and vagus
    nerve stimulation for
    depression, 90

Intensity, and electrical
    stimulation, 23

Intermittent theta burst (iTBS), 105

Internet, and transcranial direct
    current stimulation for per-
    formance enhancement, 154

Interruption-speech arrest, and
    transcranial magnetic
    stimulation, 117

InterStim therapy, 166–167

Intertrain interval, of electrical
    pulse, 26–27

Intracellular charge, 31–32

James, William, 91

Joules, 28

Ketamine, 57

KIN (potassium IN-side the cell),
    32

Kolin, A., 99

Levodopa, 122, 133

LIFUP. *See* Low-intensity focused
    ultrasound pulsation

Limbic system, introduction of
    term, ix–x

Lithium, 67–68

Location, and electroconvulsive
    therapy, 53–54

Locus coeruleus, and
    vagus nerve stimulation,
    83–84

Long-term memories, and
    electroconvulsive therapy,
    61, **62**

Low-intensity focused
    ultrasound pulsation
    (LIFUP), 170–172

MacLean, P.D., ix, 72

Magnet(s), and magnetism
    debate on therapeutic benefits
        of, **98**
    electrical current and, **18**

Magnetic field, 96, 98

Magnetic resonance imaging
    (MRI)
    low-intensity focused
        ultrasound pulsation and,
        170
    SAR limits and, 29

Magnetic seizure therapy (MST),
    55

Magnetoencephalography
    (MEG), 41–42

Major depression, and
    electroconvulsive therapy,
    64–65, 67

Mania
    electroconvulsive therapy
        and, 63, 65
    vagus nerve stimulation and,
        87

Mechanical energy, and
    generators, 19

Medical conditions, electrocon-
vulsive therapy and depres-
sion secondary to, 64. *See also*
Epilepsy; Headache; Heart
rate; Parkinson's disease;
Rheumatic arthritis; Stroke;
Surgery
Medical University of South
Carolina (MUSC), 139
Medtronic, 138, 141
MEG. *See*
Magnetoencephalography
Memory
epilepsy surgery and, 7
side effects of electroconvulsive therapy and, 61–62
test of after electroconvulsive
therapy, 52
Memory engram, 7
MENS. *See* Microcurrent
electrical neuromuscular
stimulation
Mental illness, biomarkers for,
173, 175–177. *See also* Anxiety;
Attention-deficit/hyperac-
tivity disorder; Bipolar
disorder; Depression; Mania;
Obsessive-compulsive
disorder; Personality disorders; Posttraumatic stress
disorder; Psychiatry; Schizophrenia; Treatment-resistant
conditions
Mesmer, Franz Anton, **98**
Microcurrent electrical
neuromuscular stimulation
(MENS), 168
Microtransponder, 91
Migraine headaches, and
transcranial magnetic
stimulation, 106

Milner, Peter, ix, x, 8
Mind control, concerns about in
research on brain
stimulation, 10–11, 117–118
Monoamine oxidase inhibitors
(MAOIs), 64
Morphine, transcranial magnetic
stimulation and reduction in
for pain, 114, **115**
Morphology, of electrical pulse,
24–25
Mortality
safety of deep brain
stimulation and, 131
safety of electroconvulsive
therapy and, 60, 131
Motor cortex
chronic pain and stimulation
of, 138–139
history of brain stimulation
and, 5, **6**
Motor evoked potential (MEP),
116–117
Motor stroke, and vagus nerve
stimulation, 80, 91
Motor threshold, 23, 104
Movement disorders,
neurosurgery for, 122. *See
also* Dystonia; Parkinson's
disease
MRI. *See* Magnetic resonance
imaging
MST. *See* Magnetic seizure
therapy
Multiple sclerosis, 37
MUSC. *See* Medical University of
South Carolina
Muscle relaxer, and anesthesia
for electroconvulsive
therapy, 56–57
Myelin, and action potential, 37

National Institutes of Health, 111, 143

Nerve(s), cell structure of, 33, **35.** *See also* Nervous system; Vagus nerve

Nerve growth factors, 59–60

Nervous system, and electroacupuncture, 162. *See also* Nerve(s)

Network disorder, conceptualization of depression as, 142

Neuralieve, 106, 115

Neuroendocrine abnormalities, and electroconvulsive therapy, 60

Neuronetics, 101

Neurons
effects of transcranial magnetic stimulation pulses on, 107–108
intracellular charge of, 31–32

NeuroPace, 42, 139

Neuroscience, important discoveries in twentieth century, ix–x

Neurosurgery, for movement and psychiatric disorders, 121–122, **135,** 142. *See also* Frontal lobotomies

Neosync, 106

Networks, and biomarkers for mental illness, 175

Neutrons, 14, **15**

Noninvasive cervical vagus nerve stimulation, 78–79

Norepinephrine, and vagus nerve stimulation, 83–84

Nortriptyline, 67–68

Nucleus accumbens, and deep brain stimulation for depression, 142

Nucleus tractus solitarius (NTS), 82

Obesity, and gastric vagus nerve stimulation, 79, 82, 90

Obsessive-compulsive disorder
deep brain stimulation and, 123, 142–143
transcranial magnetic stimulation and, 113

Ohm's law, 15, 16

Olds, James, ix, x, 8

Oligodendrocytes, and myelin, 37

One Flew Over the Cuckoo's Nest (movie 1975), 47

OPT-TMS trial, 111–112

Pain, treatment of chronic
deep brain stimulation for, 138–139
electroacupuncture for, 162
transcranial direct current stimulation for, 155–156
transcutaneous electrical nerve stimulation for, 160
transcranial magnetic stimulation for, 114, **115**
vagus nerve stimulation for, 91

Paired-pulse transcranial magnetic stimulation, 117

Papez, J.W., ix

Parasympathetic response, of vagus nerve stimulation, **86**

Parkinson's disease
deep brain stimulation for, xiii, 124–125, 128–131, 132–135
electroconvulsive therapy and, 66
neurosurgery for, 122

Patents, on regions of brain for therapeutic stimulation, **141**

Paulus, Walter, 148, 152

Penfield, William, 5–7, 139

Percutaneous tibial nerve stimulation (PTNS), 167

Performance enhancement, and transcranial direct current stimulation, 153–154, 156

Personality disorders, and electroconvulsive therapy, 64

PET. *See* Positron emission tomography

PFC. *See* Prefrontal cortex

Philosophy, and theory of neuroscience in twentieth century, ix

Physiology, transcranial magnetic stimulation and research on, 116–117

Polarity, of voltage, 20

Positron emission tomography (PET), and electroconvulsive therapy for depression, 58

Posttraumatic stress disorder, and transcranial magnetic stimulation, 116

Potassium, and electrostatic pressure, 32, **33**

Prefrontal cortex (PFC), and transcranial magnetic stimulation, 107, 110–112, 175

Prolonged seizures, and electroconvulsive therapy, 62

Propofol, 57

Protons, 14, **15**

Psychiatry. *See also* Clinical applications; Mental illness acceptance of electroconvulsive therapy by, 47

side effects of vagus nerve stimulation, 87

Psychotic depression, and electroconvulsive therapy, 64

PTNS. *See* Percutaneous tibial nerve stimulation

Public opinion, on electroconvulsive therapy, 47

Pulse width. *See also* Voltage effects of deep brain stimulation on brain and, 125, 128

low-intensity focused ultrasound pulsation and, 170–171

morphology of electrical pulse, 24–25, 125

Quality of life, and deep brain stimulation for Parkinson's disease, 135

Recovery, from electroconvulsive therapy, 51, **52**. *See also* Stroke

Relapse, and continuation treatment with electroconvulsive therapy, 66–67

Repetitive TMS (rTMS), 100, 103

Resistance
dosing of electroconvulsive therapy and, 48
principles of electricity and, 16, 17

Responsive neural stimulation (RNS), 126

Responsive stimulation therapy, 42, 122

Resting motor threshold (rMT), and transcranial magnetic stimulation, 110, 111
Retrograde amnesia, **52,** 61
Rheumatoid arthritis
    electroacupuncture and, 162
    vagus nerve stimulation and, 80
RNS. *See* Responsive neural stimulation
Rome, and history of brain stimulation, 3, **4**
rTMS. *See* Repetitive TMS
Russia, and development of transcranial direct current stimulation, 148

Sacral nerve stimulation (SNS), 166–167
Safety
    of cranial electrotherapy stimulation, 165
    of deep brain stimulation, 131–132
    of electroacupuncture, 162
    of electroconvulsive therapy, 60
    of transcranial magnetic stimulation, 108
    of transcutaneous electrical nerve stimulation, 160
SAR. *See* Specific absorption rate
Schizophrenia
    electroconvulsive therapy and, **57,** 65–66
    transcranial magnetic stimulation and, 113–114
Schlaepfer, T.E., 142
Scribonius Largus, 3
Seizures. *See also* Focal seizures
    chemically induced and history of electroconvulsive therapy, 46, 54

as necessary for electroconvulsive therapy, 58
    prolonged as side effect of electroconvulsive therapy, 62
    side effects of transcranial magnetic stimulation and, 108–109
    synchronous brain activity and, 44
Seizure threshold, and dosing of electroconvulsive therapy, 50, 66
Self-stimulation, and history of brain stimulation, 7–8, **9**
SenTiva vagus nerve stimulation, 78
Septic shock, and vagus nerve stimulation, 92
Sexual orientation, and history of brain stimulation, **9–10**
Shakti device, **166, 167**
Sherrington, Charles, 5
Side effects, of brain stimulation. *See also* Cognition
    of deep brain stimulation, 131–132, 135
    as different from those of conventional treatments, xiv
    of electroconvulsive therapy, 51, 53, 60–63
    of transcranial direct current stimulation, 152
    of transcranial magnetic stimulation, 108–109
    of vagus nerve stimulation, 82, 85–87
Siemens, 17
Sine wave, 52–53

Skin burns, and transcranial direct current stimulation, 152

Skinner Box arrangement, 8, **9**

Skull, resistance and conductivity in brain stimulation, 17

Sleep, and EEG rhythms, 42–43. *See also* Electrosleep therapy

SNS. *See* Sacral nerve stimulation

Sodium-potassium pump, 32, **34**

Solar panels, **20**

Sonication, and low-intensity focused ultrasound pulsation, 170, 172

Specific absorption rate (SAR), 29

Speech arrest, and transcranial magnetic stimulation, 117

Speech therapy, and transcranial direct current stimulation, 155. *See also* Aphasia

Spinning magnets, and transcranial magnetic stimulation, 106

Spiritual growth, and cranial electrotherapy stimulation, **166**

Stimoreceivers, 10

Stress reduction, and cranial electrotherapy stimulation, 165, 166

Stroke
deep brain stimulation and risk of, 131
transcranial direct current stimulation and recovery from, 154–155
transcranial magnetic stimulation and recovery from, 115
vagus nerve stimulation and rehabilitation from, 80

Subgenual cingulate cortex, and brain stimulation for depression, 139–140, 175

Substantia nigra, and deep brain stimulation for Parkinson's disease, 128–129

Subthalamic nucleus, and deep brain stimulation for Parkinson's disease, 129, **132, 133, 134**

Succinylcholine, 57

Suicidal ideation
deep brain stimulation and, 141
electroconvulsive therapy and, 65

Surgery. *See also* Neurosurgery
for epilepsy and history of brain stimulation, 5–7
vagus nerve stimulation and risks of complications, 85–86

Synaptic activity, and EEG recordings, 40–41

Synchronous brain activity, and seizures, 44

Synchrony, and EEG frequency, 41

tACS. *See* Transcranial alternating current stimulation

tDCS. *See* Transcranial direct current stimulation

Temporally interfering electric fields (TI), 172–173, **174**

TENS. *See* Transcutaneous electrical nerve stimulation

Terminology, and use of acronyms, xiv

Tesla, and magnetic field, 103

Tesla, Nicola, **20**
Theta burst, and and theta burst stimulation, 105, 112–113
TI. *See* Temporally interfering electric fields
Tinnitus
  transcranial direct current stimulation and, 156
  transcranial magnetic stimulation and, 114
  vagus nerve stimulation and, 79, 91
tLVMAS. *See* Transcutaneous low-voltage microamperage stimulation
TMS. *See* Transcranial magnetic stimulation
Transcranial alternating current stimulation (tACS), 42, 152, **153**
Transcranial direct current stimulation (tDCS)
  clinical applications of, 153–157
  effects of on brain, 149–152
  history of, 147–148, **149**
  methodology of, 148
  side effects of, 152
Transcranial magnetic stimulation (TMS)
  brain-derived neurotrophic factor and, 59
  clinical applications of, 110–118
  current research on brain stimulation and development of, xiii
  depression and, 100–101, **102,** 108, 110–113, 175–176
  effect of on brain, 106–108
  history of, 95–101
  intensity and, 23

length of train duration, 26–27
  memory and, 7
  methodology of, 101–106
  safety and adverse events of, 108–109
Transcranial random noise stimulation (tRNS), 152
Transcutaneous electrical nerve stimulation (TENS), 160–161
Transcutaneous low-voltage microamperage stimulation (tLVMAS), 168
Treatment-resistant conditions
  cranial electrotherapy stimulation for depression and, 164
  deep brain stimulation for depression and, 139
  electroconvulsive therapy for depression and, 65
  electroconvulsive therapy for mania and, 65
  electroconvulsive therapy for schizophrenia and, 66
  vagus nerve stimulation for depression and, 89
Tremor, and deep brain stimulation, 135–136, **137**
Tricyclic antidepressants (TCAs), 64
tRNS. *See* Transcranial random noise stimulation

Ultrabrief pulses, 53
Ultrasound, and low-intensity focused ultrasound pulsation, 170–172
Unified Parkinson's Disease Rating Scale (UPDRS), **134**
Unilateral placement, of electrodes, 50–52

Unipolar delivery, of electrical pulse, 27–28
University of Arizona, **132**
UroSurge, 167

Vagal block (VBLOC), 90
Vagus nerve
afferent fibers of, **83**
cross-section of, **78**
morphology of, **73**
Vagus nerve stimulation (VNS)
brain-derived neurotrophic factor and, 59
dosing of, 80–81
effects of on brain, **75,** 82–85
history of, 71–76
intertrain interval and, 27
methodology of, 76–82
Parkinson's disease and, 129
safety and adverse effects of, 82, 85–87
VBLOC. *See* Vagal block
Ventral intermediate nucleus of the thalamus (Vim), and deep brain stimulation for tremor, 135, 136

VNS. *See* Vagus nerve stimulation
Voice alteration, as side effect of vagus nerve stimulation, 86
Volt(s), definition of, 15
Voltage. *See also* Pulse width adjustments of for deep brain stimulation, 125
generators and, 20
principles of electricity and, 14, 15, 16, 17, 18

Watt, 17
Watts, J.W., **143**
Waveforms
for different forms of brain stimulation, **153**
electroconvulsive therapy and, 52–53, **153**
Weiner, Kari, 137
Westinghouse, George, **20**

Yale-Brown Obsessive Compulsive Scale, 143
Yoga, and vagus stimulation, **84**

Zabara, Jake, 72–74, 80